Ten Years That Changed the Face of Mental Illness

Ten Years That Changed the Face of Mental Illness

Jean Thuillier

English edition approved by
David Healy

Translated by
Gordon Hickish

Supported by an unrestricted educational grant from AstraZeneca

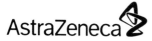

Martin Dunitz

© Professor Jean Thuillier 1981, 1999

© Translation, Martin Dunitz Ltd 1999

First published in the United Kingdom in 1999 by
Martin Dunitz Ltd
The Livery House
7–9 Pratt Street
London NW1 0AE

Tel: +44-(0)171-482-2202
Fax: +44-(0)171-267-0159
E-mail: info@mdunitz.globalnet.co.uk
Website: http://www.dunitz.co.uk

The views expressed in this book are those of the author and not those of the Pharmaceutical company or the publishers.

A CIP catalogue record for this book is available from the British Library.

ISBN 1-85317-892-6

Composition by Wearset, Boldon, Tyne and Wear
Printed and bound in Great Britain by Biddles Ltd,
Guildford and King's Lynn.

Pictured on cover (from left to right): Dr Raymond Sadoun, Professor Jean Thuillier, Dr Thérèse Lempérière, Dr Pierre Pichot, Dr Jean Delay, Dr Pierre Deniker.

Contents

Foreword   *David Healy*

Jean Thuillier is a most unusual man. He was a pharmacologist when psychiatrists had nothing to do with pharmacology, and a psychiatrist when pharmacologists had little to do with psychiatry. He enjoyed, when President of the European Society for Medicinal Chemistry, teasing these pharmacologists that their president was a psychiatrist. He was a pharmacologist and psychiatrist at the same time in a way that vividly symbolized the creation of the new field of psychopharmacology, which is described in this book.

Born in Limoges, Thuillier trained in medicine during the Second World War, taking his medical doctorate in Paris in June 1950. He began as a neurosurgeon before moving into psychiatry and into the department of Jean Delay just before chlorpromazine was discovered. He subsequently became the Scientific Director at the first INSERM unit in France in 1961.

Following his retirement from INSERM, he became the Chief Executive of a Pharmaceutical Company, one of whose products was a drug that he and his wife had synthesized and developed. During this period, from 1965 he was the founder and President of the French Society for Chemical Therapeutics, the Editor of *European Medicinal Chemistry Reviews*, President of the European Committee on Medicinal Chemistry Therapy, as well as the President of the World Congress of Medicinal Chemistry.

He began writing novels under the pseudonym of Jean Biance. The first of these published was *Bulande* in 1967. He has subsequently written books on Semmelweiss, Mesmer and Charcot. These books, as well as poetry he has written, have won literary prizes. While doing this he also opened a very successful art gallery. Truly a Renaissance man!

This is the man who tells the story of the development of chlorpromazine, the first of the antipsychotic drugs, which was the central discovery of modern psychiatry. Before its use, what we now think of as hospitals were asylums. These had degenerated into vast brutal crowded places, where a range of treatments that would now be thought of as extraordinary, such as malaria fever therapy, insulin coma and prefrontal leucotomy, were all that could be offered to patients. These had very little effect on many patients, so that for all too many death was the only release from the asylum. Many patients spent decades within the walls raving in chronic psychosis.

Chlorpromazine was the first treatment that freed these patients from their psychoses, that calmed the manic patient and indeed often relieved the burden of severe depression and anxiety. The liberation from psychosis was as dramatic as the effect of levodopa on Parkinsonian patients as described in Oliver Sacks' book *Awakenings*. Jean Thuillier describes, particularly in the case of Philippe Burg, the reawakening of a personality that is inconsistent with any use of these drugs as chemical straightjackets or simply sedatives, as critics of psychopharmacology have sometimes described them.

One of the puzzles of modern psychiatric history is why no Nobel prize was ever won for the discovery of chlorpromazine. Jean Thuillier has described, from the perspective of an insider working with Jean Delay and Pierre Deniker, the events that led to the discovery and what impact it had. In so doing he gives some insight on the play of personalities and circumstances that led to the transformation of psychiatry but to no official recognition of what had been achieved.

This book will be important for anyone with an interest in mental health, for members of the mental health profession, nurses, doctors, psychologists and others, as well as for historians of psychiatry. All too often, books on psychiatry or on the antipsychotics make gloomy reading. They tell of a terrible disease. They may tell of the benefits of treatment, but often feel compelled to discuss the problems of treatment in even greater detail. They are commonly drily technical. They may or may not be read. They are like books on Parkinson's disease, which are needed by both specialists and their patients, but equally we need books and movies like those of Oliver Sacks to give us fresh heart. And this is what Jean Thuillier's book does. This book is quite unlike any other book in that it brings a positive message that whatever problems there may be, the breakthrough has been so immense that these pale into insignificance.

There are a number of contexts that need to be borne in mind. Thuillier was writing in the shadow of the events of May 1968 in Paris, where the student revolt led to a questioning of authority of any kind. Antipsychiatry had been born during the 1960s, and nowhere was this expressed more acutely than in Paris in 1968, where the students ransacked the offices of Jean Delay. Against this background there was a compelling need to try and convey just what things were like and just what difference the new treatments had made.

It will be important therefore for anyone interested in mental health to know that from a psychiatric point of view this account rings true. Thuillier's descriptions of hospital conditions and circumstances and of the methods of treatment ring true to older psychiatrists in the field who can still remember what it was like. He populates the book with trainee psychiatrists and patients as well as senior figures and events that will be immediately recognizable to most readers of this book. He creates a world that is vivid and real in a way that could not be created by historians poring over company archives and case records decades later.

This account is important also for historians of psychiatry. There are a number of different accounts of the discovery of chlorpromazine that have been written by Judith Swazey and Ann Caldwell, as well as a volume of essays put together by Rhone–Poulenc to mark the 30th anniversary of the discovery of chlorpromazine. As befits one of the most important medical breakthroughs of the century, there should be a number of accounts, not all of which will agree with each other. Indeed one of the worrying things about the chlorpromazine story is that there have been so few accounts. In due course the events that are described here will be seen to have been as important as were the events in Vienna leading to the creation of psychoanalysis. At this time it will be important to have as many overlapping accounts as possible so that, triangulating from the various perspectives of each, it may be possible to get at just what actually happened and what the significance was of the events that took place.

Thuillier's account is particularly important among these other accounts in that it has the immediacy and understanding that comes with having been there. He tells a story with an accuracy that might be expected from a former professor of pharmacology and psychiatry. He also tells it with the panache and verve that might be expected of a man who later won literary prizes for his writing.

This is a book therefore that will appeal not only to prescribers and basic scientists but also to their families and anyone else who has an interest in mental illness. It is a gripping read that takes the reader right into the operating theatre for the first psychosurgical operation in France, introduces them to some of the first clinicians experimenting with LSD, describes some of the awful things that could go wrong, before finally introducing the antipsychotics and the antidepressants. It is rare for a psychiatric book to have an 'unputdownable' quality, but this book has just that.

David Healy

Foreword   *Ross J. Baldessarini*

The translation by Gordon Hickish and David Healy of the memoirs of Jean Thuillier makes available to English readers the recollections of a participant–observer in the truly revolutionary decade of the 1950s—the dawn of modern psychopharmacology. The book was written in 1980 by Dr Thuillier, a Parisian psychiatrist and research psychopharmacologist. It concentrates on the author's personal experiences during an unprecedented series of discoveries leading to the remarkably rapid, sequential emergence of the basic classes of psychotropic drugs in 1949–1960 that remain in wide clinical use today.

These drugs include lithium carbonate (1949), the first effective antimanic and mood-stabilizing agent; chlorpromazine (1952), the first dopamine receptor antagonist, neuroleptic–antipsychotic; iproniazid (1955), the first monoamine–oxidase inhibitor antidepressant; imipramine (1957), the first amine-transporter inhibitor antidepressant; and chlordiazepoxide (1960), the first benzodiazepine antianxiety sedative–muscle relaxant.

The book reviews a story that has been recounted several times before, and will provide few surprises to those familiar with the general outline of this remarkable series of independent and largely serendipitous discoveries. However, Thuillier's version of the story adds the strong appeal of detailed and personal anecdotes, often with the additional stylistic appeal of a mystery story. He includes many insights into personalities, their motives and interactions, and the effects of the new treatments on individuals with mental illnesses, including some colleagues.

Thuillier's view of the then-new developments from the perspective of L'Hôpital Sainte-Anne de Paris provides a clear and compelling rendition of the state of psychiatric practice at this leading Parisian mental hospital before and after the 'French Revolution of 1952'. This revolution was based on the introduction into clinical psychiatry of the first neuroleptic–antipsychotic drug, the phenothiazine, chlorpromazine. Thuillier's recounting of the first demonstrations by Pierre Deniker, Jean Delay and their colleagues of the antimanic and antipsychotic actions of chlorpromazine monotherapy at Saint Anne's Hospital is especially vivid and rich in personal details.

Thuillier himself became a laboratory-based research psychopharmacologist following clinical training in psychiatry at this world-famous teaching hospital. His forte was the use of clever animal 'models' to represent clinical disorders or, at least, to detect and objectify the effects of drugs on presumably clinically relevant behaviors. He was aided in this work by his 'green-eyed' medicinal-chemist wife and life-long collaborator, Mme Dr Thuillier.

The story introduces a cast of influential actors on the international stage who were critically involved in formalizing psychopharmacology at seminal international conferences and in research organizations aimed at encouraging research in this then-new biomedical science. Thuillier gives many indications of the rich fabric of many personal, parochial and national self-interests represented by these early players in a remarkable modern drama. The 1950s produced, arguably, the most innovative and powerful developments in psychiatric therapeutics of the millennium. The decade also opened the way to a rational, though partial and somewhat circular, understanding of the neuroscientific basis of the actions of the initial major psychotropic drugs in each class and their many imitators and variants.

Many intriguing anecdotes are provided in the book. In anticipation of the American NASA Man-in-Space Program of the 1960s, these include an intriguing and mysterious invitation by a secretive US government scientist to the Drs Thuillier to collaborate on the development of medicines that might protect against the centrally mediated shock responses encountered during extreme acceleration.

The end of the book provides a Jules Verne-like peek at a potential psychopharmacology beyond the year 2000. This futuristic vision involves frankly totalitarian psychiatric 'neuro-meddling' by computer-controlled robots and biosensors regulating the activity of surgically placed pharmaco-implants. An implication is that such technological approaches will replace any remaining vestiges of the psychoanalyst's couch. This ominous view of the future is best read for irony as an implicit warning about what might happen if contemporary techno-reductionist trends in psychiatric research and practice are pursued to their absurd extremes.

Contemporary psychiatry of the year 2000, in fact, provides a very different view from the musing of Thuillier in 1980. Although most of the discoveries of the 1950s have been greatly refined and expanded, they have not yet been fundamentally replaced. Clinical psychopharmacology continues to search for better and safer treatments, but has not recast an informed and caring physician and a patient–collaborator as central players in the therapeutic process along lines laid down in the 1950s— truly a decade that changed the face of mental illness forever.

Ross J. Baldessarini, MD
Department of Psychiatry & Neuroscience Program
Harvard Medical School, Boston, Massachusetts

'Through the influence of a purely chemical action, some substances allow man to give an unaccustomed form to the ordinary sensations of life, and to our own normal ways of wishing and thinking.'

Louis Lewin, *Phantastica*

Preface

Medicine, which is often criticized, can only be defended through a consideration of its history. Sometimes particular discoveries only reach the general public much too late, and are poorly understood because it has not been possible to explain them adequately, and because the passage of time has blurred the details and the background to these discoveries. Many branches of medicine have come under the scrutiny of authors and science journalists, who have simplified the methods used and the processes involved. The discovery of antibiotics, advances in general surgery, cardiology, cardiac surgery, renal transplants and organ grafts have so often received press, radio and television attention that everybody is now sufficiently well informed to be able—if not to evaluate and appreciate what has been achieved—at least to understand what was being attempted.

The situation is very different in the case of psychiatry, particularly insofar as its therapeutic methods are involved. It seems that people are ill at ease when confronted with this mysterious, difficult medical speciality. It must be admitted that the subject is even a little frightening. Nobody knows precisely what triggers off mental illness, and many see it as an incurable condition, which people are trying to put right with bizarre therapies, electric shocks, and now with drugs called tranquillizers.

Not only are the general public poorly informed, there are also more knowledgeable people who, in the name of freedom, have hurled criticisms and charges, as unfair as they are ill-founded, against psychiatrists and their new treatments.

Likening psychiatry to an extension of the medieval inquisition, they have accused doctors of resorting to practices more fearsome than those used then: arbitrary incarceration, electric shocks, insulin comas, brain surgery, and above all, *chemical straitjackets*. Psychiatry has been accused of drugging manic patients, of transforming violent people into terrified sheep, and rendering homosexuals impotent. 'Pharmacological brain regulation' would extend its oppression, officially encouraging the use of 'conforming drugs' with 'respectable poisons' becoming happily accepted in our social behaviour.

The truth is quite the reverse. Thanks to new drugs discovered soon after the 1950s, and to the emergence of a new branch of medicine, *psychopharmacology*, the whole face of mental illness changed within a few years. A veritable revolution rapidly transformed psychiatry and restored it to the position amongst medical specialities from which it had been excluded.

In the mental hospitals not only did the use of straitjackets disappear, but there was also a reduction in Sakel treatments (insulin comas) and psychosurgical operations, and a big drop in the use of electroconvulsive therapy. The duration of admission of mentally ill patients to psychiatric centres was greatly reduced, and a large number of in-patients were returned to an active life.

A strange paradox developed here: as psychiatric successes were accomplished, so public opinion, misinformed by partially presented facts, was inclined to think that the treatment of mental illness had gone in a direction the reverse of progress.

The truth must be clearly stated. Psychiatrists have sometimes used 'mind poisons', but only in the course of a fascinating enterprise to discover 'cerebral drugs'. I have lived through the psychopharmacology adventure—in other words, the science that has led to the introduction of the drugs of modern psychiatry. It is a story that began over half a century ago, and one that I will try to bring back to life.

J.T. (1981)

1
The snake pit

Anguish and fury

A colonel made of gold

'Sunshine in the head, sunshine in my head, to give me a different head!'
The colonel keeps repeating this as he tosses from side to side in his bed
with the regularity of a metronome. Each time I cross in front of him he
stops, sticks out his chest, stares at me, gives a military salute in my
direction as if returning one from me, and orders, 'At ease!' He adds,
'Lieutenant, go and tell Major Thomas that Battery 155 must be transferred. They cannot fire golden shells.'

Everything the colonel touches turns to gold, and with this gold he is
going to buy the world. The only thing worrying him is his head. It too has
turned to gold, and this is just not practical for him. He must find some
way of changing it, and this needs sunshine, lots of sunshine . . .

Unfortunately it is night-time, and rain is falling on Paris and the
Sainte-Anne Psychiatric Centre, a tepid drizzle, and I cannot supply the
colonel with any sunshine. His megalomaniac delirium is the result of
long-standing and neglected syphilis. The colonel is suffering from a
mental illness known as general paralysis of the insane (GPI), resulting
from syphilitic involvement of the brain. The year is 1947, penicillin has
not yet come into general use, and I shall have to 'impaludate' the
colonel—in other words to inoculate him with paludism, malaria, to try to
make his 'poor golden head' better.

That night I was on duty in the neurosurgery department, but to do my
psychiatrist colleague a good turn I agreed to cover for him on the asylum wards as well. Usually this is uneventful. However, on this occasion a
male nurse came to fetch me for an urgent 'impaludation'. I had little
experience of psychiatric techniques and confessed this to him.

'Don't worry, doctor, we'll show you what to do.' He led me to the
colonel.

'Colonel, we're going to fix you up with another head. Soon you will have
some sunshine, but in the meantime we're going to give you an injection.'

In fact, the nursing staff could have managed perfectly well without
me, but the regulations required that all therapeutic procedures should

be carried out by a doctor. I was taken to the room where the donor was waiting.

The patient lay on an iron bed, buried under the sheets, with his teeth chattering, and drenched with sweat. The instruments had been set out on a trolley, and the head night nurse showed me the temperature chart. It showed the classic textbook picture of malaria, with peaks rising to 39–40°C separated by falls—typical tertian fever, classed as benign.

'It's forty degrees Celsius—now's the time,' the head nurse told me, handing me a syringe fitted with a wide, short bevelled needle. The room was illuminated by bluish nightlights, and some other patients who had woken up came into sight. One of them called out, 'Just look at the vampires!'

As he was being told to keep quiet he added, 'Stick up for yourself, Bertrand, don't let them get your blood!'

But Bertrand offered no resistance, and just relaxed. Nevertheless the blood-taking was difficult in spite of the vein being nicely dilated below the tourniquet; for he was shivering and shaking and all his muscles were seized with spasmodic contractions. His forearm was held down on a firmly fixed board, and with luck I succeeded, after two jabs, in withdrawing ten cubic centimetres of blood, which I put in a tube containing heparin to prevent coagulation. Bertrand had watched me all the time his blood was being taken.

'He's much better,' the head nurse told me, 'and if the inoculation takes in the other patient we will stop his malaria.'

It was essential to maintain a strain of malaria in the hospital. To achieve this, the malaria-treated GPI patients were kept together in Dr Guiraud's department, and the malaria crises were terminated when a patient showed a response, but only when the protozoa had been successfully transmitted to somebody else.

I held on to my tube of blood while Bertrand was attended to, and his sweat-soaked nightshirt and bedding were changed. I was conducted back to the colonel who had been prepared by other nurses to receive Bertrand's blood. Since the two patients did not belong to the same blood group, I had to give the injection subcutaneously, and inject the whole tube of blood; whereas one or two cubic centimetres would have been sufficient if the injection could have been administered intravenously.

Transcutaneous blood injections were neither satisfactory nor reliable for an effective transfer of malaria. Abscesses tended to develop at the injection site, and the malaria crises often failed after two or three episodes. So far, everything had gone well for the colonel.

'You see, it wasn't difficult!' the head nurse commented as he took me back to the main entrance.

On the top of the main building the big clock struck three a.m. as I got back to my room, and on the tarmac of the roundabout the light of a full moon cast the shadow of the naked nymph who still frolics on the pedestal to this day.

This was the only 'impaludation' I ever performed, and indeed must have been one of the last at Sainte-Anne; for two years later penicillin transformed the lot of patients afflicted with GPI.

During this era, malaria therapy or impaludation was virtually the only biological therapeutic measure available in psychiatry apart from shock treatment. This way of treating GPI was started by the Austrian neurologist Julius von Jauregg, who had observed that the syphilitic dementias improved in association with recurrent infections, flaring up at regular intervals and accompanied by fever. Hence the idea of inoculating afflicted patients with malaria to produce tertian or quartan attacks of fever, the almost automatic repetition of which could be checked by the administration of quinine. In this way, after ten or twelve bouts of malaria, patients with GPI were observed to become calm, with remission of agitation and megalomaniac delirium. The malaria bouts were then terminated by giving quinine for five days, or by using other, synthetic, antimalarials. In thirty per cent of cases the malaria treatment improved the mental state of the patients, and some were even able to resume their professional work.

It is interesting to note that for his invention of malaria therapy Julius Wagner von Jauregg was awarded the Nobel prize for medicine in 1927, and despite all the progress achieved in psychiatry, he is still the only psychiatrist to have received this distinction.

Surgery in mental disease

I arrived at Sainte-Anne a little before the middle of the twentieth century. Having completed my medical studies apart from my thesis, I had secured a place in the new neurosurgical department that P. Puech had just set up at Sainte-Anne. Like David and a few others, Puech was a pupil of Clovis Vincent who was one of the first two French neurosurgeons, the other being Thierry de Martel. Few hospital centres were equipped for neurosurgery at the time, and designation of neurosurgeon was but sparingly bestowed by a board in Paris. It had been easier for me, training at Limoges, to be assured of designation by Puech, provided I stayed for two years in his department. It was there that I attended the first psychosurgical operations.

Patients admitted to Puech's department were mostly suffering from head injuries, road traffic accidents and brain tumours; but psychiatric work was also needed to justify the establishment of a department of neurosurgery at Sainte-Anne.

The 'mental illness surgery' was not very sophisticated. To be sure, we were no longer at Breughel's *'Stone of Madness' Operation* stage, for we worked under aseptic conditions in splendid operating theatres, but aside from cerebral tumours, which rarely gave rise to serious mental disturbances, working out ways of intervening helpfully called for a good deal of imagination.

To detect structural brain abnormalities we x-rayed skulls after introducing air between the brain and the meninges or directly into the cerebral ventricles. The terms 'intracranial hypotension' and 'cerebrovascular shock' were introduced as a basis for early efforts in what was described as 'functional psychosurgery'. Puech had around him teams of wise neurologists like Paul Guilly, and capable electroencephalographists like the Romanian-born Frenchman Fischgold. However, the true master of the department, the adviser, and Puech's source of inspiration, was Alphonse Baudouin.

This École Polytechnique graduate, eminent biochemist, neurologist, hospital physician, recently retired as Dean of the Faculty of Medicine, had been welcomed into the department by Puech and became its mentor.

Baudouin was a tall, lean man with short white hair, and pince-nez glasses which he sometimes alternated with a monocle. The stiffness of his bearing, resulting from spinal arthritis, matched his personality. His conduct during the occupation of Paris had earned him the title 'Dean of the Resistance'. His many connections and his position as permanent secretary of the Academy of Medicine gave him great authority and powerful influence—which Puech, with his eye on entry into neurosurgery, badly needed.

It was Dean Baudouin who had suggested to Puech that he should approach Jean Delay, the new professor of psychiatry at Sainte-Anne who had succeeded Levy-Valensi.

'You will gain more kudos by working with Delay, who is a physician to the Paris hospitals, than with the asylum psychiatrists,' he advised.

A collaboration was thus established with the mental illness and brain diseases clinic. A search was made for changes in cerebral structure that might underlie mental disorders, particularly atrophy of areas of the brain; 'cerebromeningeal hydrodynamic disorders' were also considered. To be honest, the research and treatments that resulted achieved little, but at least the patients were not exposed to any risks.

Time passed, and the competitive examination for Fellowship in neurosurgery was drawing near. The two principal candidates were Puech and David, and there was only one appointment available. For many months the two surgeons were building up scientific publications, each struggling to describe the rarest cases and the most spectacular results. But it was Dean Baudouin who had something up his sleeve . . .

It was a Saturday morning, at the weekly meeting, and we all assembled in the consulting room awaiting Puech. In the general discussion we were weighing up Puech's chances in the competitive examination. Suddenly Paul Guilly said, 'Look! Where has the Dean gone?'

Indeed, Alphonse, as he was familiarly known, had disappeared. The head nurse reassured us, 'He is in the boss's office.'

We waited a little longer and eventually the two men came to join us. Dean Baudouin, always stiff in his grey twill suit, walked in front of Puech who was puffing nervously at a cigarette. Puech looked worried and anxious; this was so striking that we all independently came to the conclusion that the Dean must have given him some bad news. The latter, in contrast, was imperturbable, the epitome of confidence, and he gave a discourse which was, as ever, sparkling, intelligent and authoritative. At the end of the presentation he was the first to his feet. Standing, he was taller than anyone else in the room by a good head. He leaned his straight back against a wall and slightly bent his thighs in front of Puech like Eric Von Stroheim before Pierre Fresnay in *La Grande Illusion*. Then, removing his pince-nez from his nose and stabbing the air in front of him with it like an Uhlan with a pike, he announced with a triumphant smile, 'Gentlemen, we are going to perform lobotomies!'

Lobotomy—ploughing up the brain

The subject under consideration was an operation introduced by the Portuguese Antonio Egas Moniz. This neurologist was a former student at the Salpêtrière, and subscribed to the hypothesis that morbid thoughts, generated in one part of the brain, become intensified if they are not immediately checked, so that they keep stimulating the nerve cells. He had been struck by the fact that certain kinds of mentally ill patients, particularly patients with obsessions, had a restricted psychological existence, confined to a limited cycle of ideas that dominated all others, and continually rotated in the patient's brain. This formed the basis of the idea of cutting off these morbid thoughts from their sites of resonance. Egas Moniz considered that the path from the prefrontal lobes to the thalamus (at the base of the brain) was the point at which to intervene. This was because the thalamus is the relay centre for sensory impressions, and the prefrontal lobe is where they reach consciousness. From this followed the idea of blocking this relay by dividing the thalamocortico-prefrontal fibres (leucotomy) or by undertaking partial ablation of the frontal lobe cortex (partial lobectomy or topectomy).

Egas Moniz carried out his first cerebral lobotomy (or leucotomy) in 1935, with the help of the Portuguese neurosurgeon Almeida Lima. The operative mortality was as low as one to two per cent, and postoperatively the patients were either calmer in the better cases, or else remained unchanged. The operation had not yet become widely adopted when Egas Moniz—who was a neurologist, not a psychiatrist—was awarded the Nobel prize for his work. As he was also the inventor of cerebral arteriography, I would prefer to think that the Swedish honour was in recognition of his procedure for visualization of cerebral vessels rather than his ploughing up of the frontal cortex.

However, the award of the Nobel prize revitalized this form of psychosurgery, and Alphonse Baudouin recommended that we should develop it at Sainte-Anne. He pointed out to Puech that publication of the first lobotomies in France would be sure to put him ahead in the Fellowship competition. The truth of the matter was that the Dean was curious to see the outcome of the lobotomy operation, and had struck upon a good pretext for getting Puech to go ahead. I can vouch that Puech only ever performed these kind of operations with reluctance.

I remember his anxiety and agitation the day he carried out the first lobotomy in his department at Sainte-Anne. Several times on the day before the operation, he came to see the patient, and asked him questions. He wanted to inform the family himself, and asked for their consent in writing.

In the operating theatre gallery everyone assembled to witness this 'première'. The Dean, tied up in a white gown and mask with a jersey hat on his head, took charge. The patient was laid on the table, and his shaved head was painted with tincture of iodine. The Dean himself drew the incision lines on the temples with a marking pencil, then stepped aside to make way for Puech. On each side of the skull, under local anaesthesia, a skin incision a little over two centimetres long was made, and two small retractors were positioned to ease the way for the trephine. Two symmetrical holes were bored, one above and in front of each ear; the dura—the membrane surrounding the brain—was picked up with a hook, then incised. To cut the thalamocortical fibres, Puech used a trocar—a thin nickel-steel rod—which went into the cerebral cortex as if it were butter. The direction of the probe had to be worked out theoretically, but in practice this was not very important since the excursion of the probe went right through the lobe, following two arcs each of about forty-five degrees.

Every now and then Puech moved away from his patient's skull to check the angles of the trocars from the opposite side, and this head with two steel rivets was strangely reminiscent of Boris Karloff in *Frankenstein*.

Puech, very agitated, was worried about the awareness of his patient, and kept asking him questions, which were not answered. On either side of the table a colleague and I checked the reflexes and sensation in the limbs, alert for the appearance of possible difficulties arising from the movements of the probes.

Concerned by the failure of the patient to respond to his questions, Puech shouted in his ears, 'Are you all right?' When there was still no answer, he gave the patient's arm a hard pinch. The patient made a gesture of withdrawal, crying, 'You're hurting me!' The pinch was painful—yet the section of cerebral fibres was completely painless, as is every other operation on the brain, which only has locations for integration and interpretation of pain, but no sensory receptors.

When the procedure was finished, Puech, throwing his rubber gloves down on a table, looked towards the Dean and said: 'There we are, then!'

He seemed rather worn out and thoughtful, but less worried than at the beginning of the operation. The easiness of the procedure had surprised him. In comparison with the excision of tumours, which sometimes took several hours, the lobotomy hardly took thirty minutes, with an operative time of ten minutes.

The Dean accompanied the patient back to the ward and carried out a thorough neurological examination. Everything was normal. In the ensuing days the patient experienced a little mental confusion, which quickly cleared up. I seem to remember that the original problem was an obsessional psychosis, and that this was a little improved. After the first case, Puech operated on many others—and he was the one who was awarded the first neurosurgical Fellowship.

I have stated that lobotomy was not a dangerous procedure, with an operative mortality rarely more than one per cent, but it gave rise to many noisy protests. Patients who had the operation could be divided into three groups according to the outcomes. There were those in whom the procedure produced no change and who reverted to their previous mental state. There were those who were improved, sometimes even cured—and this must be positively affirmed, for in the debate over lobotomies it would be untrue to say they were never successful; the proof of this is that they are still carried out in certain exceptional cases. But it must be admitted that there was a third category of results, where the patients were reduced to a state of 'placid phantoms', and if these patients suffered less after lobotomy, their family and friends were devastated. Perhaps anxiety had gone, and unwelcome urges with it, but at the price of lack of interest, apathy, and a flattening of affect that was often permanent.

The overwhelming drawback of this psychosurgery was that it scarred the brain irrevocably, whether the results were good, bad or indifferent; and the fact that some results were good did not make up for the bad ones. It is not a question of removing a part of the body with which one can do without, like the appendix, but of altering (certainly not every time, but very often) something essential to a human being: personality.

The Norman's voices

The foregoing description alludes to Boris Karloff and Von Stroheim, *Frankenstein* and *La Grande Illusion*. The comparisons were obvious, if a little facile—they just flowed from my pen; I am hanging on to them nevertheless, for there is something to be said for protesting at some therapeutic innovations that are merely stop-gaps from which no good can come.

So as not to dwell on a tragic or pessimistic note, nor on a delicate ethical problem, I would like to recount the story of one of the lobotomized people whose records I have kept.

He was a young Normandy peasant, very attached to his land, who had suffered all his childhood from the tyranny of an alcoholic, emotionally disturbed father, who died during a delirium tremens crisis. Heir to the estate, the patient married and had three children. He was a relentless worker, and nothing interested him except the land and what he sowed and what came up. Although well-off, he lived frugally, and his wife used to say, 'Sometimes I wonder whether he ever thinks about the children and me'.

One day he came back to the farm and without saying anything barricaded himself in his room. When urged to come out, he called out that he did not want to see his father any more. Later, following his admission to hospital with a chronic hallucinatory psychosis, his story could be put together. One morning in a field, he had suddenly developed a pain in his back, and it took all his strength to straighten his spine—all too often stooped over. As he raised his eyes, there, in an apple tree, he saw his father sitting astride a branch, ordering him about and shouting abuse just as he used to. This had never stopped; he could see his father everywhere, speaking to him and insulting him. Only thirty-five years old, he had been a compulsory in-patient for four years. A psychiatrist at Sotteville-lès-Rouen had referred him to Puech after unsuccessfully trying electroconvulsive therapy and even a Sakel treatment. With great difficulty the patient's young wife had taken over the running of the farm; wanting to try everything to get her husband better, she consented to a lobotomy on his behalf.

'The Norman', as he was called in the department, was operated upon by Puech, and apparently this was successful—so much so that when some London psychiatrists came to pay a visit it was decided to show them the patient. Given the task of making the presentation, I went to find him in his room and explained what was going to happen.

'These are doctors interested in your case, and you are going to give them your story, your childhood with your father, then your marriage and the reappearance of your father, and finally, the operation and how you feel about things now.'

I had made summaries as a framework for the presentation and explained to the Norman how I would ask him questions in front of our foreign colleagues. Everything had to go without any hitches, to give our visitors a favourable impression. Before leaving the room, I added, 'Of course, you will say how you feel now, and especially that, since the operation, you don't keep seeing your father any more.'

At this point I caught a dubious pout on the Norman's face which struck me as being odd, so I persevered, 'You do understand, the important thing is to say that you don't still have an apparition of your father following you everywhere, and stopping you working.'

The Norman didn't answer. Anxiously, I asked, 'You understand me? You don't still see your father.'

Always slow in answering since the operation, but well enough oriented and adjusted, the Norman shook his head, 'No, doctor, that's right. I don't see him any more. That's true!'

He paused, then added, 'But you see, I hear him.'

Dismayed, I stood frozen to the spot, and closed the door. In the consulting room, Puech and his visitors from abroad were waiting for the wonderful demonstration of 'hallucinolytic lobotomy'; and there was I with my good fellow who was now going to admit to auditory hallucinations. Everything was ruined, and the demonstration was going to turn into a disaster.

At the risk of losing all respect and credit from those reading these lines I will confess to the bargain I struck, and my deceitfulness. I got the Norman to sit on the edge of his bed and stood close to him.

'You remember your four years of being held at Sotteville. You know that when you leave here it will be to go home, to your farm. Your wife and children are waiting for you. You agree with this?'

'Oh yes!' he replied, with a big smile.

'Well, if you now say that you still hear your father, everything is mucked up—finished. Goodbye to the farm, your wife, your children. You'll be readmitted and sent to the asylum till the end of your days.'

The Norman seemed surprised.

'But, doctor, you haven't understood me. I told you I still hear him, but now it doesn't bother me.'

In this answer lies the essence of the good lobotomy results: lack of interest, loss of painful and distressing emotional drive from the psychological problem in question. Being a beginner in the speciality, and a sycophantic house physician to a powerful chief, instead of debating and analysing the significance of a comparative success, I wanted a complete cure. I insisted, 'You simply must not say that you can still hear your father, otherwise you'll be back in the asylum.'

The Norman understood my instructions and agreed not to mention his father's voice.

When, shortly afterwards, after I had given his history, he was asked about his hallucinations, it was with immense assurance that he replied, 'Since the operation, I don't see my father any more. He has vanished.' And turning to me he added, 'And I assure you that I don't hear him any more.'

The secret that bound us together was well kept. I saw the Norman again several times after he had gone back to his professional and family life. Everything went well and he had some more children. When he came to see me we never spoke about his father's voice. I like to think that, like his visual appearances, it must have vanished.

You will be a neuropsychiatrist

If I had practised neurosurgery in the provinces or in Paris, I would never have agreed to do lobotomies or leucotomies for my psychiatric colleagues; but in fact this difficulty never arose because the sudden death of Puech, struck down by a myocardial infarction, put an end to all my plans. Apart from Dr Brun, no member of Puech's team was to follow the career of the master, who was succeeded in his department right away by David, and later by Talayrac.

As for me, I was distraught. I went to ask Dean Baudouin's advice. I still had a year as a psychiatric house physician to do, and was signed up with Jean Delay.

'Fine; you will be a neuropsychiatrist,' Alphonse Baudouin said. He added, 'Watch and listen to what goes on while you are with Delay. He is a very intelligent man, and he doesn't do asylum psychiatry.'

This is just what the mental hospital psychiatrists had against him. In their eyes he was too much a physician and not enough a psychiatrist, too much a scientist and not enough a psychologist, too much a therapist and not enough an analyst. And anyway Jean Delay was, as they say, stuffed with distinctions: Doctor of Medicine, Doctor of Letters, physician to the Paris hospitals, Fellow of Medicine, he was at the age of forty the youngest holder of a medical clinic chair and successor at Sainte-Anne to a string of famous psychiatrists. For after Henri Claude and Laignel Lavastine, the chair of psychiatry had been awarded during the last war to Levy-Valensi, who died in deportation. To replace him, the Faculty of Medicine of Paris, unwilling to take to its bosom a mental hospital doctor, had ruled out the only valid candidate, Henri Baruk, chief physician at Charenton and a former pupil of Claude, in favour of Delay, physician to the Paris hospitals. Henri Baruk must still deplore what, along with many others, he considered an injustice. However, in spite of all the esteem in which I have always held the master of Charenton, his human qualities, his observational, symptomatological and clinical skills, and his curiosity for all biological and therapeutic problems, I believe that Jean Delay's openness of mind, his attentive agreement to any research, and his refusal to set somatic and psychiatric medicine against one another, were nevertheless very beneficial in the development of the mental illness clinic.

This was how I came to be present at Sainte-Anne at the installation of Jean Delay as professor in the chair of psychiatry, with Henri Baruk, who was his elder by more than ten years, as associate professor.

The struggle (or rather the competition) between the two men was fair but unequal; through the power of his prestige Delay got the upper hand over the admittedly exceptional personality of Baruk, who was too often baulked in his attempts to make breakthroughs. The duels lasted some time; Baruk was ready to give regular lectures at Sainte-Anne, but Delay could not bear to have ideas contrary to his own expressed in his department. (I am thinking particularly of the two men's totally opposite views on the value of electroconvulsive therapy.) Baruk had to give up his teaching sessions, and withdrew with his loyal followers to his own sphere at Charenton, where a chair was created for him and where he was to found the Moreau of Tours Society, as a tribute to the great psychiatrist and to psychopharmacology.

Sainte-Anne, a garden prison

Sainte-Anne, Charenton, Belle-Vue, Bel Air, Maudsley, Berechid . . . resonant names that sometimes cause a smile and are the butt of jokes, but also names that disturb and frighten by the images of insanity they conjure up. For in these imitation prisons inconsistency, groundless fear, overexcitement and dejection are cooped up together; and he who cannot live with anyone else because he is paralysed by excessive despair and might be driven to murder or suicide is placed in solitary confinement.

Sainte-Anne was a garden surrounded by high walls, in the fourteenth *arrondissement* of Paris, near the Santé prison, but also near the beautiful Montsouris park. At that time there was a single entrance to the hospital, along the rue Cabanis, and Jean Delay's department was called the 'Mental and Encephalon Disease Clinic'. Jean Delay stuck firmly to the 'encephalon', insisting that the word should be added, whenever anybody left it off on the pretext that it was obsolete and no longer used in texts or official documents. He was making it plain that, because his department was concerned with disorders of the mind (mental), it was natural that they should be grouped very closely with disorders of the brain and its appendages—the encephalon. He did not go so far as to say 'joined' or 'combined', but by this he demonstrated once more his refusal to bring physical and mental medicine into conflict with one another, preferring a 'holistic' concept of medicine.

Regretfully abandoning neurosurgery, I came to psychiatry with little training in this discipline, but interested in getting to know more about it and keen to help people suffering in their mind. However, it takes more than a day to understand mental illness, and the paradox of insanity was almost like a slap in the face for me. Too drilled in strictly medical science, I was entering a different world with its jargon, rituals, ceremony, and, above all, its strange therapeutic methods.

I had not entered into psychiatry through inclination, like most of my colleagues, who had frequented the asylums earlier on. My background was in medicine and surgery, and I felt disoriented in this new environment. I was first surprised, then annoyed; I had wanted to understand it quickly, and I realized that I would need firstly to watch, listen, and closely observe in order to learn to distinguish the many forms of mental illness; and above all, that I would need, as Pinel said two centuries ago, to 'live with it'.

And so I observed, listened, and lived with mental illness at Sainte-Anne, where I remained for twenty years. Admittedly I did not acquire the terminology and the self-assurance of my colleagues all at once, but soon enough I too understood that 'insanity is one man's dream, and reason is everybody's insanity'.

Two intellectual guides

Initially ill at ease in this environment of dreams, restlessness and anguish, I soon began to feel more at home through listening to two intellectual guides who dominated Sainte-Anne with their debates on the nature of insanity.

They were two friends, two comrades who I believe liked one another well enough in spite of the gulfs of incomprehension that kept them apart, and the theories they flung at one another. Great comedians capable of performing in any style, they had a high regard for each other and always richly earned ours as well. One of them, hugely knowledgeable, is famous for the sparkle and audacity of his intelligence in spite of his third-rate acting and the deliberate incoherence of his words: his name is Jacques Lacan. The other, less well known to the general public but famous and celebrated by all psychiatrists in France and elsewhere, left us some years ago. He was Henri Ey.

If I still look upon these men as two great actors, it is because they were theatrical legends. They inspired their pupils (I nearly said their public) with the passionate tone of their speech, their comic expressions, the skill of their acting, and also by the intrinsic merit of what they said, training followers of whom very few climbed up to their level. For these two great psychiatrists only inspired echoes and a few recruits from whom no fame was to come.

Henri Ey, chief physician at the Bonneval, formerly a sixteenth-century abbey, organized highly regarded symposia there that extended the Wednesday meetings at Sainte-Anne, developing and complementing them. The Wednesday meetings, started by Ey before the Second World War, were intended for preparation for the psychiatric hospitals competitive examination. They brought together psychiatrists and junior doctors and students from all areas. The Bonneval meetings were restricted to an élite, chosen by the chief, who assembled to spend several days (usually three) discussing a chosen topic. One of the most celebrated of these 'Bonneval days' was certainly the meeting of 28–30 September 1946, where the 'psychological aetiology of mental illness'—or, if you prefer, the 'psychogenesis of the neuroses and psychoses'—was discussed. In the presence of Duchène, Follin, Bonnafé, Rouart and a few others, the oratorial jousts between Lacan and Ey, which were eagerly written down, must still remain amongst the finest texts one can read on the fundamental causes of insanity.

As for me, I signed myself up more modestly for the Wednesday classes at Sainte-Anne.

Coming from his asylum at Bonneval, Ey would stay the night before the lecture in Paris, and spend the morning in the Sainte-Anne library preparing his talk behind mounds of journals and books, above which emerged his round and already nearly bald head and his powerful chest. The librarian, Madame Bonnal, had the job of deciphering his manuscripts and duplicating them. She was also the person who compiled the list of the lucky few who could go to the chief's lecture. A modest subscription was payable for access to the typed articles. The number of pages on each topic was impressive. The text was packed with places where one got out of one's depth. The references, huge and exhaustive, were well enough digested, but used in a partial manner—which was, after all, his prerogative. The lectures began in the afternoon at about two o'clock. We sat where we could, at long tables. As we had the relevant text on the subject at our disposal in advance, Henri Ey contented himself with following it rapidly, stopping to elaborate his comments. One could ask him questions, and interrupt him—but this was hardly easy. He spoke profusely, excited over what he was saying, put forward hypotheses and conclusions that he dismissed straight away, and did not hesitate to heap abuse on the great names of the present or the past.

Once the lecture was over, we moved from the library to the big clinic amphitheatre, which Jean Delay had put at Ey's disposal for the presentation of a patient. A training session was held there for the psychiatric hospitals medical competitive examination. For this, one of us selected from his wards a patient with whose records and diagnosis he alone was familiar. The patient was led on to the platform to be questioned by an examination candidate under the critical gaze of Ey. At the end of the test, the chief himself sometimes asked the patient a few additional questions, before the patient was taken back to the ward.

Then a special kind of session began, resembling a *Conservatoire* or an Actor's Studio class, depending on the atmosphere and mood of the day. The pupil on the platform had to comment on and analyse the case, and, in summing up, take the plunge by offering a diagnosis. When the pupil had finished, Henri Ey made his comments, either in agreement or contradiction with the pupil. He underlined the strong or weak points of the argument he had listened to, then, unable to resist the urge to take the stage, he took a turn at presenting the case as he felt he himself would have done at the examination. It was a delight to listen to the nicety of judgement, the analytical perspicacity, and the subtlety of some of his criticisms. We relished the demonstration of outstanding expertise. Often at the end of the class nobody remembered to open the patient's records to check the accuracy of what had been said. Ey never called for this; it was of no interest to him to verify his diagnosis; he was confident of his assessment—which in any case was virtually infallible. Even if the diagnosis had been different from his own, he would not have taken offence. So ended the show, the parade under the 'Big Top' of Sainte-Anne in front of an audience wild with admiration, which assured the great actor's success. Sometimes daydreaming at the end of the session, I enjoyed picturing Henri Ey playing Oedipus in Mounet-Sully's place, at the ancient theatre at Orange—but only after the role had been explained to him by Lacan.

In those days, Jacques Lacan was still talking and writing in an intelligible and often admirable way. I will give an account elsewhere of what I have been able to grasp from him during a session of one of his 'seminars', but I would like at this point to digress upon the value and scope of his conversation in his exchanges with Henri Ey at the Bonneval meetings, where he criticized 'organodynamism'—the famous organicist theory of insanity of the Bonneval chief. Let us listen:

> 'Insofar as insanity is the chance result of man's make-up, it is a constant feature of a wide flaw in his nature . . . Just as it threatens freedom, so it is freedom's most faithful companion, following every movement like a shadow. Not only can human beings not be understood without insanity, but he would not be a human being if he did not have within him insanity as a limit to his freedom. And just to mock this gloomy statement with our youthful humour, we can impishly note that the lapidary quote on our waiting room walls is certainly true: "He who wishes to does not go mad".'

And Lacan reached the end of his criticism using some of the humour which later became lost in the abstruseness of his talk:

> 'Having told you that Ey misunderstands the cause of insanity, and that he is not Napoleon, I end my lecture by this final proof that I do understand, and that it is I who is Napoleon.'

To which Henri Ey answered,

> 'Jacques Lacan, in himself recalling our student companionship, and in opening up again for us the magnificent screen of his dialectic, has brought back for us the happy days of our youth. At the same time, dazzled by the treasures of a psychiatry which usually keeps them hidden, we had the same disclosure of their price . . .'

And this went on for hours and days, for the whole duration of the symposium at Bonneval. To support his theories, Henri Ey, while refusing to scoff at 'naturalism', 'somatism', 'medicalism' and 'rationalism', headed in the direction of a natural history of insanity, set within the bounds of an approach that separated it from a physical cause.

> 'The thing which keeps us apart, my dear Lacan,' he maintained, 'is what sets city psychiatry against the psychiatry of the fields.'

And he added,

'In Lacan's perspective there is no novelty in the phenomenon of psychiatry. Every theory of the psychogenesis of insanity always inevitably clashes with the natural conditions causing insanity. The psychogenesis of mental illness—and Lacan is there to prove this, he will allow me to say, *ab absurdo*—like the dialectic of spiritual life, is doomed to failure. The most awful form of this failure is banality.'

He added, with a malicious smile as he looked at his comrade, who gazed back at him through big spectacles,

'It can seem that this is the word which springs to my lips after listening to this precious, substantial and musky prose from our brilliant Lacan with his style, talent, erudition and science, giving the very best of himself. Nevertheless his psychogenesis leads to the banality of insanity.'

Finally, he concluded,

'If we had to follow Lacan in his conception of psychogenesis there would no longer be such a thing as psychiatry. He has handed us its cadaver, covered with a wonderfully embroidered shroud.'

A cumbersome cadaver

Re-reading the text of these Bonneval conversations, the last sentence I have just quoted did not seem very clear to me. What was the cadaver in question? Certainly not Lacan's—but psychiatry's, of course!

I have recalled, in touching on them, what these two great men said in the 1950s to show the dialectical context in which insanity was argued over, without any attempt to find a cure. Many psychiatrists at that time were not convinced about the object of their craft. They spoke little or not at all about treatment, about therapeutic steps. It was the 'case' that interested them—the psychoanalysis of the pathological phenomenon, meticulous description, the prime mover in its genesis, and the final diagnosis. After that, they went on to another case. They would have been very surprised if somebody had said, 'Now, what are you going to do for this patient? How can we help him? What treatment are you going to give him?'

What should one make of Henri Ey's words:

'The very essence of psychiatry, its reason for existing, the origin of its position in the framework of medical sciences, the specificity of its methods, is in fact the act wherein one mind comes to the help of another mind in a beneficial meeting of understanding and rehabilitation.'

To understand, they did everything to grasp the meaning of insanity, and to explain it to others, but very few applied themselves to restoring reason. It must be confessed that the measures psychiatry had to offer were still so empirical in comparison with therapeutic advances in other medical disciplines that there was no encouragement for research.

And so physical medicine lost interest in psychiatry, which appeared a science partly concerned with 'madmen' who were mocked or feared, and which isolated itself with its jargon, psychotherapies and bizarre therapeutics. The division of the institutions, with people with physical illness being collected in general hospitals and those with mental illness in asylums, accentuated the split between the two disciplines.

It must be explained that insanity often takes very different forms.

To understand a little about mental illness

It is not my intention to describe here all the varieties of dementias, neuroses and psychoses. One book would not be enough, and it would be unhelpful and tedious for many, and of necessity open to criticism by those already well informed. Nevertheless, to help the majority understand the different kinds of medication and treatment used for patients with mental illness, I will arbitrarily classify the principal symptoms of mental illness into three paired symptom groups, corresponding to three principal kinds of therapy, in use in the past and today:

1 Mental excitation and manic agitation.
2 Depression and melancholia.
3 Delirium and hallucinations.

If you remember these three lines, you will know almost all there is to know about mental illness.

'But,' you will say, 'what about schizophrenia?' I will reply that this illness is so complex that at different stages in its development one can see all these symptoms, interlinked or alternating. If you would like to know more about it, I will tell you, like Pinel when he removed the chains from insane people, that 'to understand mad people, you have to live with demented patients so as to study their habits and personality, and follow the development of their illness day and night.' As this will not be possible, I will take you along with me to Sainte-Anne.

A morning at Sainte-Anne

It is early morning and the light of dawn shines through the fanlight above my bed. My room is high up under the roof of the Women's Baths building. It is comfortable, with a small adjoining study. But I am too close to the wards of raving patients. Every evening at sunset, for a few days, a female patient has been making a cock-crowing noise, and this goes on all night. Lulled by the yelling, I drift off to sleep, but when the noise stops at dawn, the silence wakes me up.

I go down to the ground floor to have a bath in the room reserved for severely manic women. The bathing sessions do not begin till nine o'clock and I can use the facilities before the first batch of patients. All the baths are filled at once by means of sluices operated by wheels attached to the walls. I work out the hot and cold proportions, and all the baths are filled together. I will choose one after checking the temperature.

A few weeks ago a patient cried out in her bath. She was suffering from mania, and a jute canvas had been strapped round the bathtub leaving an opening for her head. 'It's scalding, it's scalding!' she screamed. It is quite usual for mania patients to cry out, and nobody took any notice. When she was helped out of the bath, she was as red as a lobster, with second-degree burns. The cold tap had failed to open.

For me, the water is just right, and the bath very pleasant. Back in my room, I put on a pair of canvas trousers, sandals, and on top of my pullover my white coat and apron. My stethoscope! Help! The chest piece is missing! It's another of Victor's practical jokes—Victor is my white rat. I rummage in Victor's nest: a shoe box with a hole cut in the side. Under the lid, Victor is huddled up in a corner with my chest piece under his paws. I retrieve it from him. In the nest there is also a two-franc piece, an eraser, three cigarette ends, and some pieces of torn-up paper. Victor only takes paper from the wastepaper basket, otherwise it would be disastrous. I am in the process of finishing my thesis and all the pages of my manuscript are on my desk. Victor is not pleased, and follows me to the door.

'Careful, Victor, there's the cat!'

The cat belongs to the chief gardener at Sainte-Anne, and our conservatories are adjoining. One of Victor's predecessors, too keen on wandering, provided a magnificent meal for the gardener's cat, but my present Victor is a 'star' and I want to hang on to him. The spectacle of the manic patients in their bath and Victor's outbursts are the dramas that I sometimes present to my non-psychiatric medical colleagues when they come to see me at Sainte-Anne. Victor is a rat who exhibits audiogenic epileptic fits. I will explain: if I shake my bunch of keys in Victor's ears, after thirty seconds he has an epileptic fit. Truly, a proper fit, just like a real epileptic patient, with extension of the four limbs, the clonic shaking, and the coma phase. No, I am not a sadist. I am trying out some new anti-epilepsy drugs on Victor. I add a powdered chemical substance to his crushed biscuits in milk. He swallows it all, and for two days Victor has not had a fit when I rattle my keys. Ten, twenty, thirty, forty, fifty seconds—nothing. After one minute, still nothing. I can go on longer and still nothing happens. This shows that the product works.

It is time for me to go and keep an eye on my 'insulins'.

Martin's quotations

I walk along the conservatory path; the window frames are open and the head gardener is sharing out work to his assistants, selected from the long-term certified patients. Sainte-Anne is in bloom, its lawn borders neatly trimmed. In front of the men's clinic, hidden behind privet hedges, two patients are raking the path. As I cross in front of them they stop, looking at me, and one of them points a finger at me. It was he who told me one day, 'If there were more of us, it's you who would be in our place'.

Martin G. is a former teacher training college student with the top qualification in arts subjects. One day he did not come out of his room and the police were called because he was starving himself to death. After a long period of apathy and total silence, a series of eighteen insulin comas appear to have arrested the course of his illness. He started to read again, but when he was let out for a stay with his family things went badly; he slapped his sister's face for no good reason and once again locked himself up in his room. He was taken back to the hospital, and again he integrated himself into the asylum environment. Why? Nobody knows: he could not explain to me why he had slapped his sister. For many weeks, apart from sharing in the work in the garden, he is compiling a dictionary of quotations about insanity. His family bring him books— far too many books to my mind—and his greatest ambition would be to work in the Sainte-Anne library.

Martin came towards me smiling. Every day, for my benefit, he selects a quotation from those he has collected the previous day and gives me the reference. He hands me a piece of paper on which I read, 'When a madman appears reasonable, it is high time to put him in a straitjacket', and he gives the reference. Edgar Allen Poe: *Dr Gordon and Professor Plume's System*. Martin looks at me without a word, smiling. I am not very keen on these readings and selection of quotations, which are a little too morbid for my liking.

'Martin, that's fine, but I'd prefer it if you'd turn your attention to something else.'

He keeps his quotations manuscript secret. It was only much later, after a relapse followed by a lasting improvement on neuroleptics, that he told me about his compendium.

I mentioned in passing to Thomas, the head nurse, when I was in his office:

'I am not happy. Martin is not well. The compiling work is tiring him out. We'll have to tell his family to stop bringing him books. At any rate, show them to me before letting him have them.'

I had already given Martin two Sakel treatments, and during the second things nearly went wrong, so a third would be risky.

Insulin comas, still called Sakel treatments, continue to be used today, but very rarely, and only when psychotropic drugs, major tranquillizers, prove ineffective. Insulin coma was the only treatment available for schizophrenia in those days.

What *is* schizophrenia?

The enigma of schizophrenia

Schizophrenia is the most distressing, mysterious, surprising, abstruse, moving, impenetrable, disturbing and obscure of all mental illnesses. Faced with a schizophrenic patient, the greatest names in psychiatry, including Magnan, Morel, Kraepelin, Bleuler, Kretschmer, Kolman and Meyer, were perplexed, disconcerted, and eventually powerless to help the sufferer. How then can I explain this dementia, and this word which pops up almost every day from everybody's pen and lips?

Schizophrenia is psychiatry's Gordian knot, as well as being the pot in which the psychiatrist—I almost said the sorcerer—cooks all the syndromes and symptoms of mental illness. Take Marc, who has been entrusted to me so that I can look after him in the hope that one day, perhaps, he will look at the sky as you and I do, and hear the noises of the town like you and me; read, work, and talk to his wife and children as we do.

One day Marc imperceptibly became separated from the world. He became detached from his affections, his work, and friends, and all the little things of life, which now seemed empty to him. If you talk to him you will be surprised by the paradox of a mood inappropriate for the circumstances associated with an intelligence that is still fully intact. Along with his fading passions, he says extraordinary, strange, unfathomable things, using new words. His gesticulations are grotesque, but sometimes fascinating poetry emanates from his bearing and words. However, all that is but the external aspect of the inner turmoil that is dissolving his being and scouring his soul. He is caught in nets that he has woven himself, within his living flesh; you see he is alive, but his spirit is dead, or dying within the prison of the body that contains it. A stranger to others as he is to himself, his suffering is sometimes visible on his face, whilst his silence is complemented by the motionlessness of his whole body, transforming him into a statue. It is this last condition—Marc's catatonia—indifferent to food, cold and heat, that has put his life at risk. So Sakel treatments have been prescribed for Marc, to try to curb the progress of his schizophrenia.

Sakel's treatment

I knew Manfred Sakel; I met him in Paris in 1950 at the first World Psychiatric Congress, where homage was paid to him. He was a quick-tempered, arrogant man with a vicious and dogmatic spirit. He told me how he had conceived his therapy. He had been looking after morphine addicts in Berlin, at the Lichterfelde Hospital, and noticed that withdrawal caused them superexcitation, which he attributed to thyroid and suprarenal overactivity. He reasoned that an antagonistic substance could lower sympathetic tone, steady the endocrine system, and reduce the outbursts of excitation: and he chose insulin for his experiments.

In spite of the recognition that Sakel deserves for having invented the first biological treatment for schizophrenia, it must be said that his reasoning was flawed—both the premises and the conclusion.

What made him think of insulin? Banting, Best and MacLeod had isolated this hormone a few years previously and found a cure for one of the most formidable illnesses—diabetes. The Nobel prize rewarded their discovery in 1923, and everybody was talking about insulin. Faced with the lack of efficacy in psychiatry of all the medications in the pharmacopoeia, as soon as a new product was introduced in therapeutics, some psychiatrists tried it 'to see'. 'Rag-and-bone-man's work' Magendie would have called it—'they take whatever they find'. Small doses of insulin had been used to stimulate appetite in patients suffering from depression, anorexia and some chronic psychoses where the general health was severely affected. Hypoglycaemia—the lowering of blood sugar levels—produced by the insulin increased the desire and need for food. The Swiss Steck, the German Haack and the American Munn had also noticed the beneficial effect of small doses of insulin on the mood of some depressed patients.

The idea of using large doses of insulin in psychoses was undoubtedly Sakel's, but the explanation of what led him to do this seems specious to me. The truth is simpler, and more brutal. The psychiatrist who tried every new drug originating in general medical therapeutics started by administering a mild dose, then, in the absence of benefit, progressively increased the dose up to a toxic level, 'to see', and not let the chance escape of a cure by a major assault treatment—*a shock treatment*. There—the word is out: too bad! Another comparison also comes to my mind. This is the puzzled motorist whose car has broken down and all he has to turn to is the contents of his toolbox and a very sketchy technical knowledge. After a few attempts in which he has exhausted his knowledge and used all the tools, overcome by the unfathomable mysteries of the engine, despair and disarray at the failure give way to irritation, then anger. On an impulse he kicks the engine; and, *hey presto!* There is a happy surprise. The mechanism begins to move again and the engine starts.

Why should Sakel also not try to shake up the mechanism with big doses of insulin 'to see', having plenty of time after his success in inventing a fine theory. Indeed, justifying these insulin comas took some courage.

Marc's coma

The room is small but bright. Frosted glass windows filter the rays of a sun not yet very high in the sky. An hour ago Marc and Bernard were given their injections of insulin. They lie quite still and appear to be asleep in their beds. At each bedside is a nurse, and at the foot of each bed is a table covered with bottles of glucose syrup, ampoules and syringes. Everything needed for bringing them round is there, and in a corner of the room is an oxygen cylinder with a mask and regulator.

Marc's nurse gets up to check his patient's blood pressure and pulse. He says to me, in a low voice, 'I have only given sixty units of insulin this morning.' This is an adequate dose. Yesterday Marc was very difficult to wake up. It had been necessary to inject glucose intravenously whereas usually he drinks it spontaneously. Marc's face is covered in sweat, his eyes are now wide open, staring at us, but already he no longer sees or recognizes us.

'I think it's starting,' the nurse tells me.

'Starting' is our code word to mean that something is going to happen, and in this particular case that Marc is going into a coma.

At seven o'clock this morning he was given an injection of insulin, the dose being worked out in units, and in Marc's body this foreign injected insulin has begun to work. It is augmenting that normally secreted by his pancreas, which maintains the glucose—the sugar in our blood—at a constant level. Glucose is one of the main nutrients in our body, the most worthy, the most energy-providing, and the only one that our brain will accept. For brain tissue, particularly for the grey matter, glucose is essential for life and function. Under the flood of insulin poured into his body, Marc's glucose is consumed two, three or four times more quickly, like a fire in a strong wind, and Marc's liver, which usually manufactures glucose, can no longer supply it quickly enough. For a time the muscles, which, in order to work, always retain a supply of the precious sugar, give up their reserve—but soon they are no longer able to provide the quantity that the body needs, and, little by little, the glucose concentration in the blood, glycaemia as it is called, drops well below the level of one gram of glucose per litre of blood.

At first a slight thirst paradoxically accompanies copious thick salivation, then facial pallor spreads over Marc's body, which begins to perspire. His respiratory and pulse rates speed up, the muscles, which at first lost their tone, now display fibrillations, but Marc is still conscious. Without seeing him he smiles at Georges, the nurse, who maternally mops his face and chest, and changes his sweat-soaked pillow and the terry towels lining the sheets under the dressing gown in which he is wrapped. Marc is losing fluid from his organs, his skin, and his blood, in which the sugar still remaining is becoming concentrated, but nothing can slow the combustion of the glucose, and Marc's brain, deprived of its sugar, is beginning to suffer. First there are brief bouts of giddiness, and blurred vision. Everything goes pale, discoloured, and empty. Then for a few moments colours and sounds and normal vision return, a temporary improvement, which fades, the brain still struggles, but feebly, the eyes roll, the lids close, and collapse follows, with loss of consciousness indicating the first phase of cerebral impairment.

Marc, unconscious from now on, is going to need increasingly careful attention, for his coma is going to progress and become deeper as fast as the more resistant areas of the brain are affected by the progressive hypoglycaemia. He is now lying on his side, slowly moving his head from right to left; the contractions of his facial muscles, the twitching of his wrists and hands, and the sucking movements of his lips strongly resemble an suckling infant, and the comparison is apt, for, as with the newly born, it is the lower brain—the centres at the base of the brain—that is keeping Marc alive. The surface of the brain is not functioning, and only vegetative activity persists. The insulin coma has freed the lower regions from the control of the grey matter. It has created a void—an emptiness through unconsciousness—returning Marc to a level of primitive adaptation. There he is, soaked in sweat, dribbling, moaning, relatively peaceful, with absent reflexes and barely responsive to a pinprick.

The dilemma for the doctor conducting a Sakel treatment is deciding on the length of each coma: too long, and the patient cannot be revived; but, on the other hand, too short a duration represents a useless risk. Generally speaking, once the stage of deep coma had been reached, I used to maintain it for between one and two hours, depending on the pulse, blood pressure and temperature, which were checked at least every quarter of an hour, and on the neurological signs. One important point was not to reach the stage of abolition of the swallowing reflex, for the patient needed to be able to drink at the end of the treatment—I was going to say the ordeal, which it also was for the nurses. Apart from the risk of unforeseen accidents, the reassuring aspect of the Sakel treatment was that at any moment one could resuscitate, or, as we said, 'reawaken' the patient, by 'resugaring'—giving the patient some glucose syrup to drink. One or two glasses were enough to restore normal movements and consciousness, which gradually became clearer—at least to the extent that it had previously been so for the patient.

From the psychological point of view, the patient certainly came out of the insulin coma in a profound state of regression, and from then on could undergo psychological and physiological function remodelling, supported by the constant and almost maternal attention given to the patient by the medical team administering the insulin.

I have seen real affection developing between patients subjected to Sakel treatments and their nurses, and these emotional ties were important factors in the success of the treatments.

I left Marc in Georges's good hands . . .

Noise and fury

In the manic patients' ward, my arrival does not increase the tumult. Screams and shouts are the habitual background noise. The beds are quite far apart. Patients are lying down, strapped, tied up in straitjackets, feet attached to the bars of the bed with pieces of sheet to prevent bruises, and heads restrained with a halter. Patients standing, wandering about, nightshirts untied with the strings dangling. Patients shrieking, spitting, and there in the middle, three nurses, calm, good-natured, going round from one to another, tightening up a strap or untying a calmer patient. Manic patients are kept in a straitjacket if they are liable to injure themselves or another patient, but it is a strict order to untie them as soon as they are no longer a danger to themselves or to others. It is of little importance if the patient shrieks and shouts, the nurses are used to this, as they are also to cleaning up faeces and to spoonfeeding recalcitrant patients who often, laughing, spit mouthfuls of well-chewed food back into their faces.

It is in this room that I feel most humiliated by my powerlessness; I feel helpless, almost ludicrous. Schizophrenic patients may disturb and frighten me, but they are so far away from me, so indifferent to my presence. Depressed and melancholic patients disturb and sadden me with their mental suffering that deafens them to my reasoning, but I can treat them with electroconvulsive therapy and opium. But the manic patients speak to me, hurl abuse, watch me, spy on me, insult me, sing, shout and cry, and all I can do is tie them up, bind them hand and foot to their beds, give them a hot or cold bath, or knock them out for a short while with bromide, chloral or scopolamine. Put to sleep with barbiturates, the patient will be even more violent and aggressive afterwards, having found new strength during the enforced rest. In this situation the disordered mechanism is stronger than anything, and I can only wait for the end of the storm, with great care, for one cannot bathe for too long, nor tie up too tightly, nor prescribe toxic drugs in doses too strong.

How many times have I dreamt of a powerful hypnotic capable of transforming the manic patient wards into the castle of the Sleeping Beauty! But enormous doses of sedatives only had insignificant effects, and could not be repeated. We were no better equipped to cope with manic agitation than was Esquirol one hundred and twenty years earlier. Here is what he said in his famous treatise on mental illness:*

> 'If the patient's violence is extreme, he is fastened onto his bed and his movements are brought under control with a straitjacket; but he is set free as soon as he is calm again. As for those who during the day or night do not wish to stay in bed, as long as they are doing no harm, it is better to leave them alone than to constrain them.'

He was moved to pity by their fate:

> 'How many manic patients have become paralysed through being fastened too long on their bed or in an armchair!'

---

*From: Esquirol JED (1845) *Mental Maladies* (translated by EK Hunt). Philadelphia: Lea & Blanchard.

He too prescribed opium, poppy infusion, and camphor seasoned with vinegar; but also used moxa—flaming pitch put to burn on the head—or cautery applied to the nape of the neck. He added, suddenly lenient,

'You can, if you wish, substitute, for an iron heated in the fire, an iron heated in boiling water.'

I confess that sometimes, faced with certain patients who raged without respite for days and sometimes weeks, I pictured myself, as Esquirol's house physician, in desperation applying a red-hot iron to the closely cropped napes of these shrieking inmates. Only deep distress at my helplessness can excuse these unworthy thoughts.

Distress and anguish

Havelock Ellis wrote in *The Dance of Life*, 'The lunatic asylum is the place where the greatest optimism flourishes'. Naïvety, sarcasm or cruel witticism—I am not sure. However, as I left the manic patients' ward I would have liked to drag him along with me to another scene, in this smaller room, which, for some reason, seems more dismal to me, where the calmer delirium patients and the melancholic depression patients are collected together. Here the comedy of theatrical exhortations, verbal outbursts, curses and insults is no longer being performed, but instead the drama of mental suffering, phobia and obsessions, which could lead to suicide.

Frightened by life, by others, or by themselves, a vertigo had seized these other poor souls to precipitate them into anguish and despair. Formerly hellebore was administered to these pitiful victims, inconsolable depressives who sometimes have to be force-fed or they would starve themselves to death. The psychiatrist has taken the risk of using the poison of forgetfulness: opium. Like Helen pouring out nepenthe for Telemachus and his companions, patients were given a mixture of fragrant oil and opium called laudanum. Paracelsus used this name, which was applied in the sixteenth century to the viscous resin of the cist, to denote his miraculous remedy. 'I have,' he said, 'a secret substance which I call laudanum and which is better than any other remedy.' However, it was resin from the leaves and not the body of the plant that Paracelsus used, and the name is correctly applied to the opium preparation originally introduced by Sydenham. He has been called the English Hippocrates, and we also owe to him the description of the disease known as Sydenham's chorea.

Laudanum, or tincture of opium with saffron, is a preparation very rich in morphine (one centigram of morphine in twenty drops of laudanum). Melancholic patients were treated with doses of laudanum, which were increased until an equilibrium was established between their mental distress and the soothing imperturbability of opiate intoxication.

The risk of this medication was the development of dependency and addiction. So the nature of the drug was, if possible, kept from the patient, by associating it with quinine tonic wine, and the dose was reduced in stages as soon as improvement occurred. Some psychiatrists were still using laudanum when I arrived at Sainte-Anne, but melancholic depression had for several years been successfully treated with cardiazolic and electric shocks.

Cardiazolic shock

Ladislas Joseph von Meduna, director of the psychiatric hospital at Budapest, had noticed, when examining the brains of patients upon whom he performed autopsies, that the neuroglia (tissue surrounding the neurons) was very thick in epileptic patients and very thin in those with schizophrenia. He drew the conclusion from this that the two disorders must be antagonistic and that epileptic fits induced in schizophrenic patients might make them better. This is what he gave as a scientific reason when he tried later on to explain what had led him to recommend induced epilepsy in the treatment of mental illness. The hypothesis was futile, and even the existence of this thinned-down neuroglia remains controversial. In fact, von Meduna had been impressed by statistical studies that showed that epilepsy and schizophrenia hardly ever occur together in the same patient, and that a schizophrenic patient who develops epilepsy (as a result of a head injury, for example) is likely to be cured of the first illness.

First von Meduna tried camphor, then cardiazol, to provoke epileptic fits, and obtained favourable results, which were repeated by other psychiatrists, not only in schizophrenia, but also in psychoses associated with depression and melancholy. The brutality and intensity of the tonic fit, the distressing phase that preceded it, and the relative frequency of syncope and vertebral fractures soon led to the abandonment of this method. I saw it being tried out at the beginning of my medical studies by Dr Dupuytout, an eminent Limousin psychiatrist. But great credit was due to Ugo Cerletti, with his assistant Lucio Bini, for introducing the electric epileptic shock technique—electroconvulsive therapy, which is still used today with some variations under the euphemistic name 'electronarcosis'.

Cerletti's electroconvulsive therapy

Without intending disrespect to those who hold electroconvulsive therapy and its inventor up to public detraction (and I am thinking here of Henri Baruk, nevertheless always so open to all new therapies) I still have the highest regard both for Cerletti and for his method. I had the good fortune to meet him when he was seventy-three, at the World Psychiatric Congress of 1950. He was a tall, stout man, who spoke volubly but simply. He was also modest and sensitive, and only had one idea in his head, which was to find something to replace electroconvulsive therapy—'this convulsion pantomime' as he called it.

'You know,' he told me, '*nihil sub sole novi*—there's nothing new under the sun; shock treatments were discovered long before me'.

He had looked in the literature for those who had been able to precede him in his discovery, not to disparage them, but to justify himself for having been the promoter of a therapy whose procedure and technique were contrary to his sensitivities and his idea of medical ethics.

I learnt from him that Scribonus, physician to the Roman Emperor Claudius, was the first to use electricity for persistent headaches. He had a live electric ray (the fish) applied to the patient's head until the area was numbed and the pain went.

In fact, Cerletti had been interested in epilepsy since 1933. While carrying out autopsies on the bodies of epileptic patients, he had noticed hardening of the cerebral tissue in an area of the brain called the horn of Ammon. Cerletti wanted to find out if this hardening was the cause or the effect of epileptic fits. He provoked repeated epileptic fits in a dog using a 125 volt electric current. To avoid killing the animal, he only passed the current for a few tenths of a second. Meantime, he became aware of von Meduna's discovery, and tried cardiazol shock with success.

'In spite of the good results obtained with cardiazol shock,' he told me, 'the method is very trying for the patient because consciousness is not lost immediately, and it is preceded by a sensation of asphyxia which is agonizing for the patient, and for me watching his face.'

He then remembered that the electric epilepsy he had provoked in a dog was accompanied by the animal's immediate loss of consciousness, and on studying cases of accidental electrocution in the medical literature he noticed that all who survived could remember nothing about the circumstances of the accident, because of the immediate loss of consciousness once the current passed. It was thus with an essentially humanitarian objective, to prevent the distress of the premonitory phase of cardiazolic shock, that Cerletti thought of substituting electric epileptic shock.

'But I was frightened at the idea of trying this on man,' he confessed to me. 'I could not stop myself thinking of the electric chair, and of all the fatal accidents occurring through electrocution, even with current voltages so low as not to set off convulsive fits. I would never have suggested electroconvulsion if something quite fortuitous had not happened. One day an official of the Rome abattoirs told me that pigs were *killed* with electric current. And so it was to justify my refusal to use electric current in mental patients, that I wanted to be present at the slaughter of the pigs.'

'There, on a kind of stage, was a man armed with a large pair of tongs, the levers of which were connected to the town's 125 volt electric power supply. When the pigs passed in front of him, he held the two ends of the tongs, which were covered with linen moistened in salt water, across the pig's head, at the level of the ears, and immediately the animal collapsed, unconscious, immobile and stiff, like my dogs. But before an epileptic fit supervened, the slaughterer cut the immobile and unconscious pig's throat with his knife—this did not prevent the subsequent epileptic fit, which by its convulsive shaking, facilitated the flowing of the animal's blood, collected on one side for the pork butcher's shop. Thus the animal was sacrificed painlessly and in the best conditions, not by the electric shock as I had been told, but by the slaughterer's knife. With the authority of the director of Roman abattoirs, I returned to carry out experiments to try to bring about the pig's death with an electric current alone. I was then able to confirm that with a current of 125 volts, and with periods of current passage longer than several seconds, the pigs did not die, even after very violent epileptic fits.'

In March 1938, using a very simple apparatus developed in collaboration with Bini, Cerletti submitted, for the first time, a schizophrenic patient to an electric shock, and on 15 April 1938 he announced his initial results at the Rome Academy of Medicine.

The simplicity of the procedure, the total amnesia of the patient after the electric shock, and the remarkable results of the therapy in melancholic patients brought it into general use very quickly, although the outbreak of war in 1939 slowed the spread of equipment, which, with a few small variations, was always very simple. In France, after debate about the different electric currents and apparatus used, preference was given to the psychiatrist Rondepierre's apparatus, made in collaboration with Lapipe, the equipment of Delmas-Marsalet at Bordeaux being more complicated and lacking any added advantages.

For Cerletti it was the convulsive fit, not the electric current, that was the basis of this therapy, and this is why he always considered that von Meduna was the first to use convulsion therapy in psychiatry.

As for me, I have never entered the little laboratory in the men's clinic where electroconvulsive treatment is given without a certain apprehension. To tell the truth, the first electroconvulsion at which I was present did not upset me unduly, for I had seen epileptic patients having grand mal fits. But electroconvulsion, even for the most hardened doctor, was a moving spectacle, which remains today a total mystery.

The convulsion pantomime

In the room into which the sun was shining too brightly the window blind has been pulled down and we are now in semi-darkness. I am seated on a stool close to the bed. Behind me on a table a metal box measuring forty centimetres by twenty-five centimetres is connected to an electric socket. Behind the box, the lid of which is closed, there are two electric pads mounted on black handles, with their leads also connected. A large rubber strap, a short-necked bottle of salt water, a clean honeycomb-stitched towel, a syringe and needle, and some ampoules of cardiac stimulant are all ready on the table.

In front of me, the door opens. It is the first patient, accompanied by a male nurse. He stretches out on the bed after taking off his jacket and shoes, keeping on his asylum shirt and thick woollen blue trousers. This is his sixth electroconvulsion; he is calm, and looks at me confidently. The nurse, having opened the neck of the patient's shirt out widely, passes behind him, at the head of the bed, which has no headrest. Quietly he picks up the electrodes and dips the ends in the saline solution. Another male nurse, facing me, has the gag ready; he has covered the rubber strap with the towel and folded it in the shape of a pear. Meanwhile, I have opened the box and set the duration of the current and the voltage. The white contact button is ready. The first nurse lightly applies the electrodes to the patient's temples. I press the button, and the switch clock hums for a little less than a second. Less than a minute has gone by since the patient lay down on the bed.

The passage of the current is immediately indicated by a brutal contraction of all the facial muscles, in an expression like a grimace: forehead wrinkled, eyes firmly closed; his mouth slowly opens, for the tonic contraction, a true tetanus, progresses from the head towards the feet, and the neck muscles, which pull the lower jaw downwards, increase the gaping of the mouth. The nurse at the patient's head has let go of the electrodes, and supports the jaws to prevent subluxation, while the nurse in front of me introduces the rubber gag between the teeth of the still gaping mouth.

Arms and hands, body and legs, are now in extension, stretched, stiffened like wood: sometimes a cry or groan accompanies this first phase, in the course of which the diaphragm and thorax muscles, also contracted, immobilize the patient's thoracic cage so that he cannot breathe. Then a shudder, followed by a prolonged jolting, spreads over this stiff, rigid body with exsanguinated skin. At this point the mouth, as slowly as it opened, now closes again—on the gag, whose function is to push back the tongue and to protect the teeth, for the jaws contract with considerable force. Following the initial twitch, shaking develops, imperceptible initially but then of increasing amplitude. All the muscles in the body are contracting with such violence that it is difficult to imagine without seeing it. Noise from the articular surfaces of the bones as they strike against one another are sometimes audible. The two nurses are almost lying on top of the patient, weighing down his thighs and shoulders to limit the extent of the shaking and avoid subluxations and fractures. Respiration being prevented, blood loaded with carbon dioxide gives the skin of the face first a crimson then a violet hue. Finally, little by little, the shaking subsides, and finally stops. The patient is now still, limp, like a disjointed puppet. The relaxed jaws free the gag on which they were clenched, but breathing does not yet restart, and the face becomes blue-black. This goes on for another five, ten, sometimes fifteen seconds, which seem so long to me that I hold my own breath. There we are, silent, counting the interminable seconds, which creep by too slowly, and the nurses, like me, watch for the first respiratory movement, which will appear, we are sure, but which each time seems to take longer, to the point that a nurse often resorts to massage or chest compression to get it going. At last the first inspiration occurs, sudden, with a loud rattling in the throat, followed by a no less fierce expiration that brings copious frothy saliva to his lips.

This is now the third phase—coma—with muscular relaxation, and rapid, noisy breathing. The nurses and I look at one another, relieved, and already forgetting our anxiety. Everything has gone well, and the patient is moved to another room, where he will wake up again after a few minutes. In a quarter of an hour, a little hazy but quite unaware of what has happened to him, he will be escorted back to his room or to the common room. He will feel a little fatigued and stiff during the day, but that is all.

If the patient is not cooperative, as is often the case at the first session, everything is more complicated. There is a struggle, the electrodes slip, some of the current is diffused and the fit misfires. A fresh start is made, but the voltage and duration of passage of the current have to be increased almost as if a resistance had been introduced. Return of breathing takes longer, but in general everything still goes well, and anyway the patient will not remember anything.

After making the visit and supervising the treatments, my morning finishes with teaching sessions or with presentation of patients to fifth-year medical students.

From one maniac to another

This morning, Wednesday, 11 January 1950, in the main lecture theatre, I was completing the presentation of a patient who had especially interested an audience of students, normally difficult to please, who for once were refraining from munching their peanuts in front of us teachers. That day I had picked out a manic patient who was not very disturbed but sufficiently voluble for a demonstration. He had delighted everybody when he asked, pointing to the audience:

'Is it to be a film star for these kids that I've been brought here?'

I had hardly spoken. It was the patient who held everybody under his charm, telling them stories and dreaming up questions and answers. During one of these monologues, a nurse appeared at the lecture hall door, and signalled to me. Leaving the platform, where the patient went on talking, I joined the nurse.

'The duty house doctor is urgently needed in Women's Section Number One.'

I had been on call the previous day, and officially I was on duty until two o'clock, although in practice the duty stopped in the morning once the house physicians and doctors were in their departments. I was surprised, but the nurse said to me, mysteriously, 'There is trouble in the department.'

I finished the presentation to the students, and having briefly concluded the lecture, I left the lecture theatre to go to Section One of the women's department.

The patients at Sainte-Anne are divided into departments called 'open' (for free admissions) and 'closed' (for voluntary and compulsory admissions).* The closed departments are divided into sections, each with two blocks. The first block is reserved for the intensive care of acute patients and those recently admitted, and the second block houses the chronic and incurable cases. Each block is situated on one side of a courtyard planted with a few trees, and closed by a wall with a single door, which is always secured with a lock with no handle. This door is opened with a pass available to staff and the duty house doctor.

I did not use mine: the head nurse was waiting for me on the threshold. She seemed upset and annoyed.

'Dr B had an argument with Dr Abely and has hit him.'

The Abely brothers, Paul and Xavier, are both doctors at Sainte-Anne. Xavier is responsible for the admissions department and Paul, the one involved, is the senior doctor of the women's section. He is a gentle, friendly man. Standing behind his desk, he is filing scattered records and now and then wipes a graze on his forehead with an alcohol-soaked swab.

'I'm all right, but B needs some attention.'

Claude B is Paul Abely's house physician. I don't know him well. We are not in the same group, and he does not often come to the duty room. I believe he is married. Paul Abely continues, 'For two days, he has seemed excited, but I didn't know what to do.'

That morning, B arrived very early. He had come to collect the files of twelve patients in order to transfer them to an asylum in the suburbs. The head nurse asked him if the senior doctor knew what was happening, and he answered, 'No, but it can't go on like this. They must be transferred or they will be burned.'

When Paul Abely arrived, Claude B had asked to speak to him at once.

---

* There are three kinds of admissions in psychiatric hospitals in France:

(a) 'Free' admissions: the patient asks spontaneously to be in hospital. These patients can leave when they like, and nobody can prevent them.

(b) 'Voluntary' admissions: patients are admitted at the request of their family or a friend or relative. They can leave at the request of their family or a third person who takes responsibility, but only with the approval of the doctor, who can decline if it is felt that the patient is not cured.

(c) 'Compulsory' admissions: made by prefectorial order in *départements* or by the Chief of Police in Paris. Release is only granted by the administrative authority on the recommendation of the doctor.

'I've chosen twelve women who must go. You must sign their transfer.'

When Paul Abely asked him the reason for this decision, he first refused to answer, then exploded, 'So! You too are in league with the Inquisition. But your Inquisition sentence will not be carried out. These women will not be burned. They are not witches.'

He grabbed the office lamp by its base and banged it hard on the table. The glass shade, as it shattered, injured Paul Abely's forehead. Claude B then panicked, and ran away to shut himself in a room on the first floor. The senior doctor did not want to publicize the incident; he knew that B had had a previous attack two years earlier.

'It is up to us to do something, but as his aggression was directed at me, I cannot take part in this personally, and above all I cannot keep him in a closed department.'

He asked me to admit him for a time to the free department of the clinic, and I agreed. But difficulties began: I had to persuade him to follow me, of his own free will, for I did not want to have him transported in a straitjacket on a stretcher.

Claude B's witches

In the room where he had taken refuge, Claude B soon took me to task.

'Who sent you to judge me? Who do you think you are? Torquemada? The secret court is not for me . . . '

I tried to give an answer, but couldn't find the words. I sat down near him on the edge of the bed, and for a moment, side by side, we kept quiet, without moving. Eventually I got up.

'Come and rest in my department—I have an empty room. You will be by yourself.'

It took me some time to convince him. Grandiosely, he said, 'There are those who get rid of their mad patients through courts, asylums, prison, and now, once again, as in the days of old, funeral pyres are being got ready.'

I tell him, 'You'll tell me all about this soon. Let's not stay here. Come with me.'

In the end, he agreed to follow me. He had kept on his white coat, and in the corridors nobody paid much attention to these two doctors who walked along talking. For B continued to hold forth:

'Centuries of celibacy, you hear? Centuries of celibacy have not inhibited the clergy's erotic urges. Now the priests want to get married. Women excite men's passions. They are possessed by the devil, they are witches who must be burned.'

A whole sarabande of demoniacal ideas danced in Claude B's head. He had read the Inquisitors Jakob Sprenger and Heinrich Krämer's *Malleus Maleficarum*, the *Hammer of Witches'*, the treatise on exorcism and pornography that codified the execution of heretics and mentally ill people, described as witches, in the Middle Ages.

'I assure you. It's coming back. There used to be subterranean passages between the monasteries and the nuns' convents. They are starting again.'

He had proof that the priests in the church in the rue de la Tombe-Issoire came looking for madwomen at Sainte-Anne every night, coming through the catacombs.

'They manage to get them out, and they burn them like witches.'

He stopped, rooted before me, marking his words with expansive gestures, holding onto my sleeve. People passing by looked at us, surprised by Claude B's rather agitated chatter, but as I appeared to be listening attentively to him, they merely saw an animated conversation. I took him by the arm to lead him on, and he continued, 'You know what they do to them, the witches, before making them appear before their judges? They shave their genital organs so that the devil cannot hide in the pubic hairs.'

He started to laugh, slapping his thighs. I could not stop myself from asking him where he had found Sprenger and Krämer's book.

'At the Nationale. A translation by Montague Summers.'

I managed to turn the conversation to the library at Sainte-Anne, and he began to criticize the classification and the glossaries of the books.

A hundred metres at the most separated the mental illness clinic from the Women's Section, and we spent more than a quarter of an hour covering them, with B's pauses and dissertations. Once in the room prepared for him, he stretched out fully clothed on the bed, looked at me in silence for some time, and then said, 'Put me to sleep.'

For some time Dr Guiraud, senior physician of the second Women's Section, had made use of the hypnotic properties of a synthetic antihistamine, promethazine hydrochloride (Phenergan), to calm agitated patients. Unlike chloral, barbiturates and other more toxic drugs, which cannot be given for too long, doses of promethazine could be repeated without trouble. This particular use of promethazine by Dr Guiraud must be pointed out, because chemically this drug belongs to the phenothiazine group, which gave rise to chlorpromazine (Largactil), the first great medication in psychiatry. I gave B an injection of a hundred milligrams of promethazine and he quickly relaxed. A few days later, he left the department to go to a private clinic.

This adventure of my colleague has remained firmly marked in my memory, because of another dramatic happening the same day.

From one drama to another

In spite of discretion being brought to bear on B's hospitalization, some people knew about it, and during lunch in the duty room one of us remarked, jokingly, that we must beware of any contagion, that we didn't play enough, and that we needed a 'tonic'. A duty-room 'tonic' was a sumptuous and very boozy dinner, to which outsiders were welcomed as guests—these were often artists and people from show business. We enjoyed mingling with a different crowd, laughing at the difficult circumstances of the times.

As steward in charge of supplies, it was my responsibility to provide the food, guests, and drinks for these meals. We arranged the food with the hospital kitchen chef; the manageress of a bar in the rue Washington assured us of a recruitment of guests; and wines and spirits, which were still in short supply, were taken care of by our colleague L.

'Where has L got to?' somebody asked.

I do not know whether I will be believed, but what matter! Perhaps it was fatigue from the night on duty, and the stress of the long time spent talking with B, on top of the day's work, but at this particular moment I had the vision of L stretched out on a deserted beach. Why a beach? I followed up my idea, recalling a Brittany shore in an enclosed bay where fishermen were dragging nets on the sand. I was far from the questions which were being exchanged around me, about the absence of L, who had not been seen for three days—Sophie T had asked for him several times. Instead, I was on this beach where fish were being hauled in, and L was amongst the fishermen.

L was discreet, spoke little, and was particular about his food. He drank water—only ever water—even at our 'tonics'. He went to his uncle, who had stores at the wine market at Jussieu, for the wines and spirits he obtained for us.

'We must go and look in his room.'

It was Lucie Laure who said this. We knew about L's love for Lucie Laure; an entirely platonic love in spite of L's attempts. I took L's spare key from the bunch of keys in the duty room. His room was in a dilapidated part of the Sainte-Anne building called the 'cells', which were none other than the old individual cells of the manic patients' quarters. The management had joined them together in pairs, to make reasonably comfortable resident's rooms, opening on to a little green space, the remains of an old walking area for the insane.

I tried to open the door; the key turned in the lock but the door was obstructed by a chair. We all pushed together. The handle gave way and we went in.

L lay in blue pyjamas on his unmade bed, with his head turned towards the bedside table, where there was a letter, beside a glass of water and several tubes of barbital.

Behind us, Lucie Laure remained in the doorway, looking very pale. We made the gestures and reactions to be expected in the presence of our friend's body. These were moments I remember poorly. In my memory, they are veiled in mist. Of my visions of the beach, the fishermen, and the shore where I had seen L, all that now remained for me was the atmosphere of this hospital, of this tragic scene, of too much fear and anguish, and too many tormented souls. Here, everything irrational seemed normal. Every question was answered in vague terms that were used without being understood.

Claude B's crisis, and L's suicide, overwhelmed me. I had the feeling of having been drawn into an ambush. In spite of all the zeal I put into learning about psychiatry, what I was doing did not satisfy me. I had chosen to learn medicine to provide care and to cure. What I had learnt in nearly ten years did not help me at all in treating mental illness. The therapies I was using had no scientific basis. I was a powerless onlooker at illnesses for which I could only offer the assault of shock treatments.

Besides my colleagues who had come into mental illness medicine out of choice, and who stoically endured agitation and delirium, there were others who through access to mental illness had sought to resolve their own illness, and like Claude B and L had succumbed in the attempt. Although I felt in no danger of sharing their fate, I had become desperate to escape. That is why, for the last year, I had been going regularly every afternoon to work in the pharmacology laboratory of the Faculty of Medicine. It was again the Dean, Baudouin, who obtained this opportunity for me. I had been to see him to tell him about my disappointment and disillusionment. I told him about my approach to mental patients and the spectacle of my daily drama.

'The sight of mental illness is terrible,' he said to me, 'but the description you give of it is even more frightening. You exaggerate and you are not fair. Before curing, you have to know what you are dealing with. Now you are learning.'

He added, 'I have something to ask of you. Find me a few epileptic patients at Sainte-Anne. I have a preparation to try out—this will be a diversion for you.'

A few days later, I had compiled a list of ten epileptic patients. I went back to find the Dean and explained the cards on which I had entered the kind of fits and their frequency. An experiment could be started.

'Fine,' said the Dean. 'Now we are going to get the preparation from Hazard.' And he took me to the professor of pharmacology.

A laboratory smelling of sulphur

The rabbit's electric shock

The laboratories of the pharmacology department were in the rue de l'École-de-Médecine, in the Faculty premises. I remember being struck by the pervading smell when we entered. It was a mixture of unusual odours, the components of which I subsequently learnt to analyse, but in which sulphurous smells predominated. We were in an organic chemistry laboratory. The Dean announced his arrival, and Professor René Hazard came to meet us. He was a thin, dry little man with a bony face and prominent red cheekbones; he looked tiny beside the Dean, to whom he showed great deference.

His little office was installed in an understairs cupboard between two laboratories. He told us to take a seat, and called in two colleagues whom he introduced to us. One was the head of the organic chemistry laboratory, Pierre Chabrier de la Saunière, who was interested at the time in sulphur drugs, and the other was his co-worker, Jean Cheymol. The Dean said that, thanks to me, he had found ten epileptic patients and that the 217 HC clinical trial could begin. The letter 'H' was Hazard's initial and 'C' that of Chabrier, who had synthesized the product—perhaps also Cheymol's, who had studied the substance in animals. The index '217' was the number of the entry in the laboratory record book.

After a short account of the product, René Hazard handed over to Chabrier, who drew some formulae for me, and explained the syntheses and the introduction of sulphur into the molecule. I didn't understand this very well, any more than Cheymol's explanation about the toxicity of the product. Pharmacology was in those days inadequately taught. Students learnt by heart the doses of prescribed medicines, and took no interest in their mode of action. As for chemical formulae, I can state that not one doctor in a hundred would have been able to write down the formula of aspirin. I looked attentive, but I only heard with half an ear what was said to me, till suddenly a sentence surprised me. Cheymol had just said '... and 217 HC has a remarkable action on electroconvulsion in the rabbit.' For me, electroconvulsion conveyed images so far removed from the little mammal that I wanted an explanation.

Jean Cheymol was too serious a man to play with rabbits! He gave them electric shocks to provoke an epileptic fit, as I did in humans. This was not to change the morose frame of mind of the little animal, but to induce experimental epilepsy. In this way he produced what is known as a pharmacological 'model', resembling the disorder of epilepsy, on which he could study antidotes, 'anti-epileptics'. He had given his rabbits 217 HC in a sufficient dose, and although given electric shocks they subsequently no longer developed convulsions.

With René Hazard's agreement, Jean Cheymol allowed me to be present at his experiments. I was especially interested because this enabled me to follow all the stages in the development of a drug right through to its trials in humans. I saw 217 HC synthesized in Chabrier's laboratory, and its toxicity studied and its effectiveness confirmed on rabbit epilepsy models.

Up to this point I had never been concerned about how drugs are made and what stages are gone through in the course of their introduction. One thing, however, had struck me even in the first years of my medical studies: doctors who chose the medicines for every illness, and alone had the ability to prescribe them, were not those who discovered them. It was in pharmaceutical product laboratories that discoveries were made, under the direction of pharmacists who in theory do not know about medicine and illnesses. Doctors prescribing, pharmacists inventing: it seemed strange to me that it should not be the doctor, being in contact with the illness, who should find the medication. This problem is in truth much more complex than it appears, and deserves an analysis, which perhaps I will make one day.

I noticed that all the workers in the pharmacology laboratory, with the exception of the chemist Chabrier, were pharmacists. Admittedly Hazard and Cheymol, both hospital pharmacists, were also doctors, but they had studied medicine after pharmacy, as an addition, without fully understanding it. In learning pharmacology and the essentials of pharmacy with Jean Cheymol and René Hazard I was only completing and deepening my understanding of medicine, whilst in studying medications which they could not and dare not try on humans, they themselves remained merely pharmacists.

So every afternoon I went to the pharmacology laboratory; first out of curiosity, then as an attentive pupil. The problem of epilepsy interested me considerably. Jean Cheymol was a conscientious scientist and an excellent operator, who taught me all the appropriate techniques for provoking epilepsy in the rat, the rabbit and the mouse. As well as electric fits, we made use of chemical fits not only with cardiazol, but also with strychnine, picrotoxin, and thujone, which is present in absinthe essence. It was also possible, in some selected rats, to provoke epileptic fits with a loud noise, or even by shaking a bunch of keys in their ears for a sufficient time. And so, little by little, the very practical pharmacology that I practised in the afternoons provided relief after my all-too-psychiatric mornings.

This complementing of clinical psychiatry with pharmacological work fascinated me, and I felt privileged to have a foot in each discipline. I had also noticed that epilepsy makes a bridge between medicine and psychiatry by the use made of the convulsive fits, and the therapeutic research to which epilepsy gives rise. I was to find another point of contact as well, another intermediary between pharmacology and psychiatry: this was the eternal problem of alcohol.

Alcoholism and psychiatry

Alcohol overdosage, a social phenomenon leading to chronic alcoholism, brings people who are endangering themselves or others to the psychiatric hospital. Acute alcoholism, bouts of delirium tremens, as well as psychosis and alcoholic dementia, are all manifestations of mental illness with an obvious toxic cause and with simple and effective treatment, at least for earlier cases.

The person with alcoholism is, in the asylum population, the patient with the best prognosis, and the in-patient who will be the soonest free. Should I confess that I was glad to welcome them into my department? After the acute phase of delirium tremens, in which unfortunately life was sometime threatened, progress towards a cure happened quickly with effective treatment. Depressive or angry drunkenness, whether or not complicated by confusion, hallucinations, serious character disorder, or even psychosis, improved with alcohol withdrawal, and were cured with correction of eating habits, and the prescription of lipotropic factors and vitamins. The 'wino' made a good patient, quickly dried out and cured. But the problem remained of consolidating this good result through appropriate re-education. One knows how little credit must be given to the pledge of the drunkard who, lax by nature and no longer supervised, begins to drink again.

Certainly, alcohol 'deconditioning' treatments have been tried, establishing conditioned reflexes of disgust in the alcoholic patient at the sight of drinks. Little use was made of these methods, which were complicated to apply, until the day when the anti-alcoholic action of disulfiram (Antabuse) was exploited.

Antabuse

Like many discoveries, that of the anti-alcoholic action of disulfiram was a chance event, but came about through careful observation of new phenomena, and identification of the cause by intelligent scientists. I obtained the strange story of his discovery from Erik Jacobsen himself.

In 1948, Jacobsen and Jens Hald, pharmacologists at the Medicinalco Pharmaceutical Company in Copenhagen, were studying new vermifuges. They found that certain sulphur-based products combined with the worm's blood to form toxic compounds capable of killing the parasite. One of the most active of these compounds was tetraethylthiuram disulphide, which we will refer to for simplicity as 'Antabuse'—the name chosen by Medicinalco. The Antabuse molecule contains four sulphur atoms; very toxic for parasitic worms, but hardly at all for humans.

Jacobsen and Hald took some Antabuse to confirm this absence of toxicity, and also to rid themselves of worms which had infested them in the course of their experiments. Still under the influence of the medication, they each had to be present at separate receptions, where they drank some alcohol. They suddenly had to retire to bed, with a strange set of symptoms. A few days later they were relating their misadventures to one another. The symptoms experienced were identical: bright flushing of the face and neck extending to the chest and arms, ringing in the ears, a rapid pulse, headaches, giddiness, nausea and drowsiness. They studied the phenomenon in detail, and suggested using this unpleasant Antabuse–alcohol reaction to bring about a distaste for drink in people with alcoholism.

I had read Hald and Jacobsen's first scientific publication in the British medical journal *The Lancet*, which we had in the Faculty library, and I remember showing the article the same day to Pierre Chabrier, who, as I have mentioned, was very interested in sulphur drugs.

'This product can be made very quickly for you,' he told me, and introduced me to one of his students, Germaine Nachmias, who was writing a thesis for her doctorate on products closely related to Antabuse. She agreed to interrupt her personal work, and in forty-eight hours made 200 grams of Antabuse for me.

In those days the strictness of the Public Health Ministry requirements regarding the control of drugs had not yet reached the constraining and research-discouraging level that it has today. Within a few days, the pharmacology of Antabuse was worked out; in two weeks the tolerance and toxicity were being tested in animals, and twenty-three days after my reading the article in *The Lancet* the first patient began treatment with Antabuse in Jean Delay's department at Sainte-Anne.

A year later, on 20 June 1950, I presented my Doctorate in Medicine thesis entitled 'Pathogenic and therapeutic trials in alcoholism. Research on Antabuse'. For the first time, a psychiatrist and a pharmacologist sat side by side to preside over a thesis undertaken jointly in their two departments. Jean Delay and René Hazard, who only met one another on Faculty boards, talked that day about psychiatry and pharmacology. Hazard had undertaken to question me on the pharmacology of Antabuse, which I had worked on in his laboratory, and Jean Delay on the observations and clinical results obtained with psychiatric patients in his department at Sainte-Anne.

This thesis was possibly one of the first psychopharmacological theses, before the term had been coined, more perhaps because of the collaboration of the two disciplines that I had brought together than because of the subject of the thesis itself.

I have to say that the word 'psychopharmacology' was not uttered at any time, and the unusual juxtaposition of the two men I had brought together would certainly not have led to effective cooperation, so much strangers were they to one another. Instinctively, psychiatry frightened Hazard, and animal experimentation was repugnant to Delay.

As for me, I still did not foresee on that day the importance that psychopharmacology was going to assume, nor that the brunette with big green eyes who had made the Antabuse for me would accompany me in this venture.

The psychiatrists' fair

On 19 September 1950 the first World Psychiatry Congress opened in Paris. At the instigation of Henri Ey, who was its secretary-general, all countries except Germany were officially invited, and delegates arrived from throughout the world. It was a gigantic fair, a psychiatric 'celebration of mankind', attended by psychiatrists and psychoanalysts from all shores, of all beliefs, friendly or rival scientific societies, and lawyers and psychotherapists. The Congress reports, edited the following year, took up more than a metre on library bookshelves.

Henri Ey set up his congress as one would the Olympic Games, with national committees in which all sectors of psychiatry with their disciplines were represented. As is customary with Congresses of the Association of French-Speaking Psychiatrists, each session had its reporters and discussion guests, the meeting being followed by paper sessions on the subject involved.

If Henri Ey as secretary-general was the kingpin of this imposing display, the presidency of the Congress could go to none other than the holder of the chair of psychiatry in Paris, Professor Jean Delay. Mindful of protocol, but with little interest in the practical problems and (it must be said) incompetent at organizing a congress, Delay, although consulted regularly by Ey, left him to it. He restricted himself to putting some of his pupils on the organizing committee to make sure that his school's authority would not be diminished.

A ceremonial address

The inaugural session of the Congress took place on Tuesday 19 September in the great lecture theatre of the Sorbonne, where Jean Delay was to give the welcoming address to Congress participants.

Although every French person present and most foreign delegates were already familiar with Henri Ey and his works, a mystery hung over the medical knowledge and psychiatric competence of Jean Delay, only recently appointed as professor of the mental illness clinic at the age of forty. Mostly known in Paris, Jean Delay's personality had not yet attained the fame and prestige which it was to earn from the first day of the Congress. In fact the address he gave remains a masterly account, and a successful attempt to sum up the state of psychiatry in 1950. Leaving no aspect in the shade, analysing trends, theories and methods, speaking just as well about biology as about psychoanalysis and therapy, giving his judgement on every point, the lesson was clear, the historical relations correct, and the presentation dazzling, in the most flawless dialectic style. Finally, with the most elegant sophistication, juggling with names, references and dates, which he detailed with exactitude and precision, Jean Delay spoke without any text or notes, and held his audience spellbound, under the charm of his address, for over an hour. Opposing the two philosophies of reason and intuition, he painted a panorama that ranged from Descartes and Pascal to modern medical psychobiology.

He also recalled the first international psychiatry congress of the century—that of 1900—which was confined to the classification of mental illness and could only take note of the relentless advance of most psychoses. He then commented:

'In 1900 Magnan said of the Paris psychiatry congress, that it was the Public Assistance congress. Now, in 1950, this congress must be positioned under the sign of therapeutics, fruit of the efforts and progress of all human sciences from the biological sciences to the moral sciences between which psychiatry fills the intervening gulf.'

He concluded, 'If the word cure, so serious because of the hopes to which it gives rise, must only be pronounced with reserve, it is no longer forbidden to us.'

The great psychiatrists of the time responded to Jean Delay's address with prolonged applause. Then a marathon of reports, discussions and papers followed. If psychoanalysis held the place of honour, in spite of the absence of Freud, who died in September 1939, the spotlight was on the section devoted to shock therapies, where Manfred Sakel, Ladislas von Meduna and Ugo Cerletti climbed on to the platform to describe their work, and to receive great praise or violent criticism. Indeed, this congress was far from reaching a consensus on the solutions proposed for all the problems discussed.

Panegyrics and rebukes

Chronologically, Sakel treatment (insulin coma) had been introduced in 1927, cardiazol convulsion therapy in 1929 and electroconvulsive therapy in 1939. Sakel, von Meduna and Cerletti made their contributions in that order.

Sakel spoke extensively, recalling his initial hypotheses, the state of the psychiatric services in 1927 in Berlin and especially in Vienna, and the purely philosophical and psychological 'jargon' of the psychiatrists. He gave a masterly description of Otto Poetzl's department in Vienna, where he had been allowed to carry out his first insulin comas. Proudly, he recalled that his method had been the first to be called 'shock therapy', and that Cerletti and Bini, before introducing electroconvulsion, had been consulting him since 1933 to inform and educate themselves. He only spoke about von Meduna to say that his technique had contributed little, and that, in contrast, he himself with insulin had achieved an eighty-six per cent cure rate in schizophrenic patients whose illness was of less than a year's standing. Manfred Sakel, arrogant and dogmatic, brutal in his words, scornful even of his colleagues, provoked a mixed reception from the audience. Von Meduna, whom he had offended, conspicuously refused to shake hands with him. By its tone, Sakel's report cast a shadow of discredit on a man who had nevertheless found the first valid treatment for schizophrenia.

Von Meduna was much more modest; he recognized that before him George Burrows, in England, had used camphor to treat a case of mania by producing convulsions. In response to Sakel, he said that the large number of comas that were irreversible, and the dangers of insulin therapy, had been the sole reasons behind his desire to find a more practicable and less dangerous treatment. He also spoke of a technique he had just begun to use: 'carboshock', which involved producing convulsions by the inhalation of a mixture of thirty per cent carbon dioxide and seventy per cent oxygen. Patients breathed this mixture for 30–120 seconds, to induce a fit. Twenty to fifty sessions were needed, at a rate of three per week. In practice this procedure was subsequently little used.

Much more human and likeable than Sakel, von Meduna was more freely applauded, even though cardiazol treatment (as he pointed out) was indisputably less effective than insulin in schizophrenia. The greatest ovation, however, was reserved for the man who had invented electro-convulsive therapy, a method that nearly everyone present agreed to recognize was effective and relatively harmless in manic-depressive and melancholic psychoses. Ugo Cerletti deserved this tribute all the more because this great doctor combined simplicity and moderation in his words with huge dignity, winning over all the Congress participants.

Cerletti began his talk by speaking of von Meduna, of his convulsion therapy technique which he differentiated from the convulsions of Sakel's treatment, which were of quite another kind; and perhaps to compensate for the unfair things said by the latter about cardiazol therapy, he said to von Meduna:

'You were the first, with your method, to draw my attention to the therapeutic effect of convulsive fits, and today I say "thank you" to you.'

He then sketched a panorama of the whole history of electricity in medicine. After recalling the earliest origins of electrical therapy, including the use of electric rays for migraine in AD 45, he spoke about the Leyden jar, Franklin's condensers, and of Volta electrifying men holding one another by the hand, of Leduc using his famous 'electric current' to induce sleep in 1898; of Batteli who, in 1903, had produced the first epileptic fit in a dog, putting one electrode on the nape of the neck and the other on its nose. I was especially surprised and interested to learn from the inventor of electroconvulsive therapy that Jean-Paul Marat, our Montagnard National Convention member, famously stabbed by Charlotte Corday, had been doctor to the Count of Artois's guard in 1776 and that he had used electric current to 'stimulate the health of the young recruits'. He had even published a paper that had attracted Franklin's interest.

After recounting the steps that had led him to use electroconvulsive therapy and which I have already reported, Cerletti gave details about his technique and his apparatus, set up with Bini, and the current used: 120 volts for a tenth of a second. He made it clear that with the electrodes placed on the temples, little current reached the chest and abdomen, and that there was no risk of it reaching the heart, as happens if the electrodes are positioned on the ankles, wrists and on the head, for electrocution in the electric chair. 'Each of us,' he said, 'has hidden in his brain a ready-made wiring diagram for an attack of epilepsy. But a detonator is needed, and the threshold must be reached for a fit to take place.'

This therapeutic fit, which according to the speaker left no aftereffects, acted on the diencephalic region (at the base of the brain), where the centres for mood regulation are situated. He provided his success statistics, rightly specifying that his method was basically the treatment of manic-depressive psychosis.

Finally, Cerletti showed us a film he had made demonstrating the development of epileptic fits in all kinds of animals, from fish to humans. 'I've made this film,' he told us, 'to show you that in all species of animals, including man, the epileptic fit is accompanied, wherever it occurs, by an intense fright which strikes them dumb and paralyses them, and that all the convulsions which shake them afterwards resemble a defence reaction. I know very well that the electroconvulsed patient, like the epileptic, has no memory of what happened before the fit, and that amnesia is complete. But I have always felt embarrassed, ill at ease, and even seized with remorse before the "convulsive pantomime" of major epilepsy. I remember having told my assistants, after the first electroconvulsion success, that the method must sooner or later be got rid of, and mankind must be spared from electroconvulsive therapy. Yes, gentlemen, I confess to you, this was the first thought which came to me when I carried out the initial electroconvulsion on man. Alas, we are not yet there.'

He ended by saying that he was working continually in the hope of being able to say one day, 'Gentlemen, electroconvulsion is no longer practised; we have found the substance, the medication, which is taking its place.'

Pacheco e Silva from São Paulo, who presided over the session, thanked Ugo Cerletti for his talk and told him of the recognition that doctors and patients owed him for a form of treatment which was effective in nearly seventy-five per cent of cases.

The floor was next given to the participants for free discussion. Immediately the opponents of shock treatments declared themselves, and one of the most virulent was Henri Baruk. Straight away declaring his opposition, he spared the speakers neither sarcasm nor denigration. Far from giving them credit for their therapeutic success, he presented the results in a specious manner, and, redoubtable quibbler that he was, pleaded in the name of morality and non-violence. For him, it was brutal treatment, breaking bones, and violating the moral personality because it was carried out without the patient's consent. 'These practices must be condemned and forbidden,' he maintained, 'all the more so because manic-depressive psychoses improve and get well on their own.'

This point of view of Baruk's, who had few supporters, was not that of the majority present. Most, while recognizing that they were ill at ease over convulsions, the therapeutic mechanism of which they did not understand, were in agreement in recognizing their favourable results in cyclothymia, manic-depressive psychoses, and in stuporous forms of schizophrenia. Some, like Juan Lopez Ibor from Madrid, who presided over the discussion session, after questioning one another about mental personality and psychiatric therapeutics in general, agreed to say that electroconvulsive therapy was no more brutal than the surgeon's knife, that its dangers were minimal, and that it was difficult to make patient consent a necessary requirement since the patient was not always in a fit state to give it. As for Georges Heuyer, hospital physician and famous tribunal psychiatric expert, he considered Baruk's position frankly unacceptable, reckoning that, 'Shock treatments have radically transformed the lives of these unfortunates, and it is not right, in the name of a demagogic moral doctrine toadying to squeamishness, to wait weeks, months or years for a hypothetical cure.'

He added, 'In a country where a tax on balconies has always been rejected as a violation of the right to air and light, to repudiate effective therapies claiming them to be an attack on the human personality is to weigh down the mentally ill with chains yet again.'

Kalinowski from New York, Muller from Munsingen, Wohlfarth from Stockholm and Ziskind from Los Angeles also took part in this memorable discussion.

The session devoted to psychosurgery and lobotomy was likewise attended by an audience that was attentive and critical, but less impassioned, for authoritative opinion already considered this procedure, which caused irreversible damage, to be only a stop-gap. Amongst those performing this operation, Sargant from London defended it in cases where the precision of the indication had given him verifiable successes.

The congress at play

However, the 1950 World Psychiatry Congress was not solely confined to reports about shock treatment. Psychiatric nosology (the description and classification of illnesses), the psychological or organic origin of mental illness, psychological testing, psychiatric institutions and, of course, psychoanalysis, were also discussed.

Sigmund Freud had died eleven years earlier, and many of the psychiatrists attending the conference had known him, either at the luxurious apartment he occupied in Vienna, at 19 Berggasse, surrounded with antiques and oriental rugs, or in the simplicity of the little cottage in Hampstead, in London, as a refugee from the Nazis.

His memory was celebrated at the Congress, but already dissident doctrines had many disciples. One such was Alfred Adler, who rejected the practice of sitting behind the patient lying on the couch, believing instead that a direct face-to-face conversation was needed, and that psychotherapy was essential.

As for Carl Jung, who had contributed in such an important way to the spreading of Freud's ideas, he attracted particularly those who, like him, did not accept the master's sexual ideas and his concept of libido.

The austerity and severity of the working sessions gave way each evening to artistic and cultural occasions. Each night brought a new diversion. So the Renaud-Barrault Company, the Roland Petit Ballets, the Conservatoire concert orchestra with André Cluytens and Jeanne-Marie Darré, Tabarin, Lili Bontemps, and Juliette Greco's French cancan were all applauded. The Louvre's doors were opened for an evening with a buffet in the antiques galleries. And as for the closing banquet, this was held in the foyer of the Palais de Chaillot, facing the floodlit garden fountains.

In order to make the Congress official, on Thursday 21 September Vincent Auriol, President of the Republic, received delegates from forty-six countries, presented by Jean Delay, at the Elysée.

Exhibition pictures

The general public was also to take part in the event. Leveillé, director at the Palace of Discovery, had given permission for an international exhibition of the history and progress of psychiatry, which filled several rooms. Fourteen nations participated in this exhibition. A synopsis of all the important steps in psychiatric knowledge, from the earliest times to the present day, was represented in the form of paintings, illustrated plates and reproductions. Museums had loaned famous works. Pinel could be seen setting free mentally ill patients at the Salpêtrière, with the help of his senior nurse Pussin, and in the presence of National Conventioner Couthon, as could William Tuke and his family founding their famous free retreat for the mentally ill in York. Also seen was the Italian Vincenzo Chiarugi, who, in 1788, three years before Pinel, set up a free psychiatric department at the Bonifacio hospital. Gabriel's famous drawings were on show, depicting the different types of mentally ill patients described by Esquirol in his treatise. The public could also assess, in two rooms, the therapeutic progress of a science seeking to show that it was also medical.

I confess to being perplexed over this endeavour, for what was on display resembled measures for stating the question rather than methods of treatment. Innocently, the person responsible had thought he was doing well in explaining everything with the help of sketches, photography and even anecdotes. Cardiazol, insulin and electric shocks were described. There were diagrams showing how lobotomies and lobectomies (excision of cerebral cortex) were done, how general paralysis of the insane was cured with impaludation in combination formerly with arsenicals and now with penicillin; thermal fits produced by sulphur-treated oils, and short-wave radiation which made the patient's temperature rise to over 40 °C were referred to. Even the instruments used for these treatments were on display: Lapipe and Rondepierre's electroconvulsive therapy kit, and that of Delmas-Marsalet, and the lobotomy knife belonging to Fiamberti, who operated as the patient lay on his bed after an electroconvulsion.

I was left wondering, since the Palace of Discovery's function was to popularize science, whether, as with chemistry and electricity, demonstrations of electroconvulsions and lobotomies could not be offered free to the public!

In the final section of the exhibition was a secluded corner set aside for medicinal therapies. Jacobsen's anti-alcoholic Antabuse, the amino acids prescribed for retarded people, glutamic acid, and a new product used by Delay and Deniker called Suxil (about which I will speak later) were put together in an ill-assorted manner. In this isolated cul-de-sac, notice boards referred to psychochemistry, and to relationships between mental equilibrium and moods. Since I was known to work with pharmacists I had been asked to check that the chemical formulae drawn by the Palace's graphic designer were correct. At that time—and to this day, what's more—even if they had been wrong, no psychiatrist would have noticed!

2
Preludes

An unusual menagerie

The World Psychiatric Congress in 1950 ended on an enthusiastic note. Despite the mixture of ideas and the customary psychiatric verbosity, a few doctors had expressed an interest in finding medicinal therapies for mental illness. This gave me encouragement to persevere in joint pharmacology and psychopathology research.

I had been appointed assistant to the pharmacology chair, and I directed a research laboratory at Jean Delay's, which worked in liaison with the mental illness clinic. This was, I believe, one of the first psychopharmacology laboratories.

A 'hideous cookery'

Whether sensitive souls like it or not, before trying a medicine on humans, it must be tested on animals. Medicine only makes discoveries in so far as it is spared the harassment and unfair rumours that so often paralyse it. The criticisms of animal experimentation are mostly baseless. There is no longer any vivisection. All operations are performed under anaesthesia. Outside laboratories it is certainly possible to find sadists and perverts who torture animals, but scientists are not among them. When Claude Bernard was asked if anybody had a right to experiment on animals, he replied unequivocally:

> 'I think one has this right, completely and absolutely ... it is only possible to rescue living beings from death after sacrificing others. I do not accept that it would be moral to try more or less dangerous or active remedies on patients without having tried them initially on dogs.'
>
> He added, answering unjustified criticisms: 'After all, should one be moved by cries of sensitivity, or by the objections which men who are strangers to scientific ideas have been able to make? All sentiments are respectable and I will be careful never to offend any. I explain them clearly and that is why they do not stop me.'

But Bernard recognized also 'that it was not easy, in the middle of the cries of animals, and flowing blood to work in a horrible charnel house ... to follow a nerve ending in livid stinking flesh which would be an object of disgust and horror for every other man . . . ' He concluded with resignation understanding the science of life could only be achieved by a ghastly 'cookery'.

The 'cookery' I tried to do was not easy, for if pharmacology had few recipes, psychopharmacology then had none.

It is possible to study a diuretic drug by measuring the increase in urine volume of a dog, a cardiac tonic by observing the action of the product on the contractions of a rabbit's or a frog's heart. One can measure the depth and length of sleep produced by new hypnotics in rats, mice, even fish. But how can one study a drug that calms the mind, that tranquillizes, quietens down fits of rage, clears away hallucinations? Animal patients are needed to whom the illness has been transmitted, to study possible therapies.

It was certainly known how to induce epilepsy, how to infect mice, rats and guinea pigs with bacteria, and transmit rabies, cholera and poliomyelitis to dogs, chickens and monkeys; but how could mania and melancholy, hallucinations and phobias be transmitted to animals? Before giving a newly formulated agent to a patient, one needed to know if it was calming or excitant, if it was likely to act in agitation or depression, and if it had some chance of reducing anxiety or anguish.

Experimental neuroses in animals

It is known that animals can be trained to carry out tasks which they perform regularly when they hear a sound or see a signal. It is also known that this sound or signal, if repeated, can also set off a reaction in the animal called a 'conditioned reflex'. The Russian Pavlov identified the rules of this 'classical conditioning'. The American psychologists, particularly Thorndyke, Watson, and especially Skinner, did even better—they created what is known as 'operant conditioning'—which I am going to explain while simplifying it to the extreme.

There is a cat in a cage who is hungry. He sees before him a wire mesh box containing food, which he cannot get at. He paces about in the cage, trying unsuccessfully to open the box. After this has gone on for a while, the cat inadvertently puts his paw on a lever on the floor of the cage; the food box opens, and a piece of meat slides out, which the cat can eat. After a period of training, each time the cat is hungry, he will press a lever and obtain a piece of meat. Everything is fine: here is a cat taught to press on the lever, and rewarded for his common sense. But now the nasty scientist intervenes. Our satisfied, happy cat continues the game: one paw-push on the lever, and each time, a piece of meat; once, twice more, and then suddenly, no more meat—instead, a powerful jet of ice-cold air makes Minet jump, and he takes refuge in a corner of the cage. So at each push on the lever there follows, haphazardly, sometimes a piece of meat, sometimes the blast of cold air. After a while, Minet no longer knows whether he is destined for the carrot or the stick when he presses the lever, and rather than try any more, he will give up the effort.

Crouched in the corner of the cage, his coat bristling, an anxious look in his eyes, jumping at the least noise, the cat is transformed into an anxious creature, sometimes even aggressive, mewing without reason and without conviction. The reflex of pushing on the lever remains to some extent; one sees a paw reach out but it is withdrawn at once, and despondency and weary immobility return, in spite of hunger.

Using this method, neurotic, anxious, psychologically ill cats can be produced, whose behaviour is an exact replica, and an almost perfect model, of an anxiety neurosis. On this anxious cat, the ingenious investigator will try out a selection of drugs and mixtures so that the patient can see the world through rose-coloured spectacles again.

Therapeutic intoxication

Having produced a neurotic cat, the problem remained of finding a product that would make it forget the cruel dilemma of the piece of meat and the current of air. When I used this method for the first time, before the discovery of neuroleptics and tranquillizers, nothing worked. I tried products that increased the animal's fright and others that plunged it into a state of torpor from which it emerged only in an even greater panic. Two mixtures, however, did make my cat forget the diabolical box: one was a mixture of barbiturates—phenobarbitone (Gardenal) or amylobarbitone (Amytal)—and amphetamines (psychotonic products which prevent sleep); the other was a beverage made from milk and alcohol. In the case of the first treatment, the animal seemed to perk up, comforted, walking boldly towards the box and trying, in spite of the current of air, to catch his mean sustenance; but quickly discouraged, he resumed his sullen attitude and made no more attempts. It was more difficult to get the cat to accept alcohol-laced milk; however, by starting with little doses of alcohol, gradually I transformed Minet into a drinker who not only enjoyed his drink but gradually preferred his mixture to pure milk. Then it was a jovial drunkard who entered the cage, played with the lever, got a jet of cold air in his nostrils, but shot out his paw to grab hold of the box. Rolling onto his back, belly and paws in the air, he again made several attempts that brought him a long-awaited reward or an inconvenience that left him unconcerned. This phase of euphoria faded, to disappear at the same time as the alcohol vapours, and after the stage of intoxication the reality of the conflict and the anxiety reappeared. So I found with my alcoholic cat the same way of evading problems as all those who seek oblivion at the bottom of a glass of alcohol.

The creation of experimental neuroses in the cat called for enormous amounts of labour and patience, and significant results were too few to meet the need to test out many therapies and chemical products. I needed to have a large number of animals, above all more practicable than our domestic cat, who is not always easy to handle.

I have hesitated to describe these researches in 'experimental psychiatry', which may disturb some people, but since I have taken Claude Bernard as an advocate, I shall continue my story, sheltering behind his speech in defence of experimental medicine.

Yes, animal models resembling human psychoses and neuroses, and mimicking insanity, are necessary in order to try out medications capable of counteracting mental illnesses. Subsequently the biochemistry and mechanisms of action of these drugs were studied to find others, but before these first discoveries, nothing was known. It was not known whether depression or excitation was expressed by diminution or increase in brain activity, by specific neurosecretions. One had to feel one's way. And along this narrow path, I walk in the footsteps of my neurotic cats, my spiders, my turning mice . . .

Murderous rats

There are rats who can live peacefully with white mice. There are others who are killers of mice, and to pick them out there is only one way—to put the animals together.

Here in a glass cage is a white mouse nibbling a biscuit; a rat is placed near it. It has been picked at random from a batch of the same strain. First surprised, it remains still in front of the mouse, which continues eating or busies itself with various comings and goings, indifferent to the intruder. The rat may adopt two different attitudes: either it remains calm and peaceful, and tolerates the mouse—or it breaks the back of its neck with one bite. This 'assassination' can happen very soon after the two rodents have been put together, or some time later.

Some killer rats attack the mice in less than two minutes, while others cohabit peacefully. We needed to know if the assassin rats could be rendered inoffensive by the use of medication. In 1951 no product had yet been discovered capable of overcoming the murderous instincts of these animals. However, one could pacify these assassin rats by putting a fine needle into their brain and injecting atropine into the lateral part of the hypothalamus, and conversely, by injecting carbachol in the same way, peaceful rats could be made into killers. Atropine is an inhibitor and carbachol an activator of cerebral acetylcholine, the substance that normally controls impulse transmission in our nerves and brain.

I had managed this very delicate operation more or less successfully thanks to Horsley-Clarke's apparatus, enabling the needles to be guided into the exact area where the injection had to be given. I operated following landmarks determined from the rat skull anatomy. I noticed that my interventions made the rats calmer, even apathetic, when they did not die, but I did not believe in the specificity of action of chemical substances directly introduced into the brain. In reality the trauma caused by the operation was alone responsible, and the results were directly related to the functions of the zone that were stimulated or destroyed. I also noticed that when I left the needles in place in the rats' brains, some appeared particularly active, while others, as I have indicated, sank into a torpor when I removed the needle.

These observations were to find confirmation in the work of the American James Olds and the Spaniard José Delgado, who implanted electrodes into the brains of rats and delivered electric currents in different areas to modify the animals' behaviour. They noticed that the rats appeared to derive pleasure from the sensations they perceived, to the point that if a device was made so that they could stimulate themselves, they operated the lever that sent the current several hundred times an hour.

These methods allowed me to pick out the animals on whom I would try new drugs. However, these rats were fragile, and difficult to find. The operations involved were long and delicate: this is why we looked for other procedures, methods and actors with whom to work.

Siamese fighting fish

The *Betta splendens* male or Siamese fighting fish is a fine aquarium fish with long handsome caudal fins of glistening colours: iridescent red, blue and yellow. Alone with one or several females it is peaceable, but if two males find themselves together, a merciless struggle takes place until one of the two adversaries is killed. With fins spread out, in glistening colours from full dilatation of the chromatophores that carry the pigments of the scales, the two combatants attack each other without respite, tearing out scraps of one another's fin and skin with their sharp-edged mouths, aiming particularly for the reproductive organs and swim bladder. This model of aggression lends itself particularly well to the study of drugs, which can be added to the aquarium water. I noticed that calming substances always made the brilliant colours of the Siamese fish turn pale, and they then became colourless at the same time as indifference and loss of aggression developed, so that the two former enemies could move around in the same aquarium.

Thus did I set up, at Sainte-Anne, a strange menagerie of neurotic cats, killer rats and aggressive fish; but for my colleagues who came to visit my laboratory, two particularly unusual attractions were suggested: my turning mice and my trained spiders.

The IDPN turning mice

Although researchers with microscopes had never been able to detect any difference between a normal brain and that of a schizophrenic patient, wiser biochemists found that some nerve cells have greater activity than others, and that the metabolism of some cellular nuclei could be stimulated with chemical substances. In this way two Swedish scientists, Holgar Hyden and Artelius, had shown that in certain conditions malonic dinitrile could modify the structure of the neuron (nerve cell). They also tested this product and its analogues on handicapped brains.

Experiments were carried out at Sainte-Anne in this direction, looking for active 'dinitriles'.

I had learnt that a young researcher, J.-P. Marquiset, who worked with Professor Delaby at the Faculty of Pharmacy was preparing a thesis on substances related to the nitriles. To synthesize the substances of his thesis, he had to produce intermediate products, which mostly were dinitriles. Marquiset let me have eleven dinitriles, which I immediately undertook to study.

Before every experiment with a drug on an animal, it is necessary to determine the margin existing between toxic doses and minimal active doses; this is called calculating the toxicity of the drug. To do this, one has to deliberately kill animals to find out the minimal fatal dose, beside which the action of the product can be studied. I did this with the eleven dinitriles from Marquiset, injecting them into mice. Of course, the mice did not all die, and I kept the survivors in a cage. Now, a few days after these studies, I witnessed in this cage the strange sarabande of two mice who, in the middle of their fellow creatures, had made a trail for themselves along which they ran relentlessly. It was all the more striking that the other mice, perhaps surprised or even frightened by the two agitated ones, were crouched, immobile, in the corners of the cage. I isolated the two hot-headed creatures in a glass bowl where, after a moment, they began running around again. Stopping only to feed, these turning mice also slept at night—and even in the daytime—but if they were touched, after a few disorganized gambols, the circular race began again, uncontrollable, for hours. The energy used up by these little animals was enormous; their considerably augmented metabolism was balanced by a commensurately increased food intake.

The spectacle of these mice, running round at such a lively pace, was staggering. I could not stop myself from comparing their incessant whirl with the unrest of agitated patients. I foresaw the possibility of using this agitation to test sedatives and tranquillizers, but I needed to be sure that this hyperactivity was persistent, and above all to understand its cause.

Determining which of the eleven dinitriles provoked the 'waltzing mouse' syndrome took me more than a month; and I set aside several weeks to work out the dose that reliably set off the phenomenon. Once the investigation was finished, I was able to present the report on my work to the Biology Society.

This was the first time that *permanent* excitation accompanied by turbulent agitation had been induced in an animal using a chemical substance. Certainly, with caffeine, amphetamines and some nitrate derivatives, animals could be excited for a short while—but only during the period of action of the substance. As the medication was eliminated, the agitation ceased. However, my mice, after one single injection, began to become agitated from the second day and were running round on the third: furthermore, this agitation continued until the death of the animal, which occurred within the same time limits as the average length of life of mice. Since the product that provoked this agitation syndrome was iminodipropionitrile, I called the animals 'IDPN turning mice'.

These IDPN mice, which could easily be produced, were studied not only in my laboratory but also in many other research centres, and gave rise to a large number of experiments. I used them mostly for selecting and assessing the action of different drugs. They also enabled me to check and confirm Jean Delay's classification of psychotropic drugs, and to separate central nervous system depressants into three groups: neuroleptics, drugs for psychoses; tranquillizing sedatives, drugs for neuroses and minor psychiatric disorders; and hypnotics, drugs for attention and sleep disorders.

Some disappointed hopes

The discovery of the permanent excitation syndrome of the IDPN mouse had given birth to hopes in all those who had followed the work of my laboratory. The chemists thought they had produced an original substance that could have therapeutic applications; the clinicians, myself included, dreamed that this dinitrile that agitated the mouse so well could perhaps break the deadlock in patients with catatonic schizophrenia, and bring part of the asylum population out of its torpor. We were to be disillusioned.

The molecule responsible for the syndrome, iminodipropionitrile, was a dinitrile of the base that was used to produce the other ten compounds. There was nothing original about the chemical formula; it was a derivative of the acrylic nitrile used in the manufacture of plastics. It could not be patented.

As for clinical applications of the product, there was already the risk of creating a lasting permanent excitation in human subjects, but above all, the lesions I had observed in the cerebellum and base of the brain of these mice forbade any therapeutic application. However, some researchers who came to study the turning IDPN mice in my laboratory suggested that perhaps very small doses might have a stimulant effect on cerebral metabolism without producing lesions. I never decided to try, for small doses were ineffective in the animal, and permanent lesions appeared suddenly as soon as a threshold dose had been exceeded.

The chemist Marquiset, to whom I explained that IDPN was unusable in humans, accepted this with regret, but Professor Delaby never understood why Jean Delay and I did not have the courage to try the product. I never managed to convince him, and he has a grudge against me for this refusal. However, apparently none of the other scientists who used IDPN—and there are many of them—ever dared to go on from animals to humans.

The star and his impresario

I had made an apparatus for the turning mice to measure the components of their agitation. I thus obtained graphs and charts for studying substances that worked on the animal. One single category of products were calming, the hypnotics, but at the price of a heavy sleep. A few minutes after the injection of a barbiturate, the turning became uncoordinated, the animal staggered, then lay down on its side and sank into a semi-coma from which it rose after ten minutes to resume its running again. I had an exact replica of what happened with agitated patients treated with phenobarbitone. The same thing happened with promethazine.

These results, which I had reported to the Biology Society, attracted many comments and questions, but I was especially pleased by the compliments of one man whom I have always held in high esteem, Professor Jean Roche.

Jean Roche, who had first taught biology in Marseilles, was professor at the College of France and secretary of the exclusive Biology Society. A biochemist specializing in endocrine physiology, he was a man of rigorous reasoning who at the Biology Society accepted only precise work, supported with evidence and with concrete results. I was full of apprehension when I presented myself to give a talk about my observations; when I had spoken earlier about my mice to the pharmacologists Cheymol and Hazard, I had been greeted with amused scepticism, rather than interest. What is more, Hazard had ironically remarked, 'One of your stories of lunatics again.' He had never taken my attempts to create models of psychopharmacology seriously. When I showed him my mice and the film I had made about this excitomotor syndrome, he had pointed his finger at me: 'Careful! Pharmacology is not performed with circus acts!'

I had been vexed, and his remarks cast doubts in my mind about the value of what I had discovered.

As for Jean Delay, he did not understand; not that he could not, but because all animal experimentation got under his skin. As he rarely came into my laboratory, I had taken a mouse into his study, where it started running round. He had got up quickly, saying to me, 'Fine! Thank you. I've seen it. Take it away!'

He had, however, added, 'What does Hazard think about it?'

He wanted his colleague's back up. I answered, 'He said that it is extraordinary.'

I had told a lie; it was Jean Roche who had said this to me, when congratulating me after my presentation to the Biology Society.

When the text of my communication appeared in print a few months later, I received a large number of letters, many from abroad. I was overjoyed to receive one from Professor Ernst Rothlin of Basle, scientific director of the Sandoz Laboratories, who invited me to present my mouse before all the scientists of his company.

A journey to Basle

This trip to Basle was a memorable one for me. The friendly welcome from Ernst Rothlin, the great scientist, the unprecedented luxury of the Swiss laboratories compared with the poverty of our French university hospital facilities, the meeting with Albert Hofmann (the discoverer of lysergic acid diethylamide, LSD), the discussion that followed the showing of the film I had made about my mouse-star, and above all the interest of a great pharmaceutical company in the kind of research I was pursuing, were the first worthwhile encouragement for my work.

Rothlin, to whom we are indebted for important work on rye alkaloids, and who developed Hydergine (co-dergocrine mesylate) which brought great wealth to Sandoz, had foreseen the scientific and commercial interest that could arise from the discovery of medication for the psychoses. This was why he was interested in everything going on in this field, and why he had strongly encouraged his assistant Aurelio Cerletti and the chemist Albert Hofmann in pursuing their work on hallucinogenic drugs.

Another surprise was waiting for me at Rothlin's laboratory. Before showing me to the conference room where I was to give my talk and show my film, I was taken to visit a magnificent aseptic air-conditioned animal house where I was introduced to 'Rothlin's waltzing mice'. These were waltzing mice, running round like mine, but running round genetically, selected from tens of thousands of Sandoz's mice and born with this characteristic. Unlike my IDPN mice, which gave birth to normal mice, Rothlin's waltzing mice produced mice that also turned, albeit in small numbers. Rothlin recognized that my procedure had the advantage of being able to provide as many turning mice as desired.

My journey to Basle made me acquainted not only with two men who became my friends, Rothlin and Hofmann, but also with the Basle pharmaceutical industry, its luxury, scientific and technical quality, and the spirit of emulation that inspired it. I had been encouraged by scientists who, like me, were interested in therapeutic research into mental illness. I had also become certain as a result of this contact that this kind of research was not utopian. And it was with great confidence that I returned to Paris with many ideas and hopes in my head. I also had two grams of LSD in my pocket, which Hofmann had given me; enough to make more than ten thousand people take leave of their senses.

Héloïse's webs

Before my meeting with Albert Hofmann, I received some LSD from the Sandoz Laboratories through the post; a few centigrams in a cellophane packet slipped into a letter. I used it for experiments on animals, and on humans as well. The two grams which I had been given constituted a supply that would last me for a long time. At the moment I only had one taker for this product, and this was my spider Héloïse.

I had read in the scientific magazine *Experientia* that the biologist P. N. Witt used spiders to study hallucinogens, and I too wanted to use this approach. With many difficulties, I found some spiders able to spin webs at a good rate, to faithfully repeated designs and geometrically well constructed. The species used by Witt were not available in Paris, and I had to fall back on a breed of spiders that the head of the Vivarium laboratory had introduced into the Jardin des Plantes.

Snakes, salamanders, insects, lizards and toads were imprisoned in cages, but the spiders would only spin their webs if they were completely unconfined, and that was at the bottom of the building where they had an overheated room, in the middle of which a desiccated bay tree, planted in a sand pit, spread its dead branches. The spiders made their webs between the tree and the angles of the walls.

They were large *Nephila* spiders from Madagascar, with bodies as big as a small nut and long, chitinous black-and-orange legs. Their web is so strong that they can capture birds, and the thread they spin has been woven into fabric. They were fed on big white worms (flour worms), which were thrown alive onto the web.

The boy who had the job of looking after the spiders picked one up and it stayed still in his hand.

'They are not harmful,' he told me, 'or venomous. Sometimes they bite, but this doesn't hurt any more than a bee sting.'

I was not completely reassured by these words, any more than by the necessity of keeping them at liberty. I went back several times to the Vivarium to get used to handling these creatures, but it was not possible to carry out my experiments in the Jardin des Plantes; the substances I wanted to administer to the spiders presented too many risks for the precious and rare animals in the Vivarium. Very kindly the director agreed to make me a present of a spider. I chose it from amongst those who spun the most beautiful webs, and as the laboratory boy who raised them was named Pierre Abelard, I baptized the chosen one Héloïse.

When I arrived at Sainte-Anne with my spider I stirred up an outcry in my laboratory. The fish and the turning mice were well accepted, and even considered entertaining; the welcome for the neurotic cats and assassin rats was more reserved; but Héloïse, in spite of her name and the beautiful colours of her legs, inspired nobody. When it was learnt that she had to have a place where she could roam at liberty I received a delegation from the hospital staff who told me politely but firmly to stop this sort of experiment. I acquiesced, but with the complicity of Dupin, my laboratory boy, I put Héloïse in the animal house between two rabbit cages.

The next morning, Dupin came looking for me, dismayed. Héloïse had disappeared. We looked for her unsuccessfully for several days. Then one morning we were overjoyed to discover, stretching between the handle of a window in the animal house, the ceiling and the wastewater drainpipe, a magnificent web, of perfect geometry, and with the hub of the trap nicely centred. But still no Héloïse: she was sulking. I had a supply of flour worms, and I threw several onto the threads of the trap, where they remained stuck and wriggling. No doubt hungry and attracted by the delicacy, greedy Héloïse came out from between the bars of a rabbit cage and began her meal.

Héloïse, having paralysed her prey, sucked out all the contents, putting the digestive juices needed to liquefy all the organs into her victim's body. I had the problem of giving her my hallucinogens as well. There was no question of giving her injections, which would have wounded or killed her. I had succeeded in training Héloïse so that I could hold her in my hand, but she refused to eat there. To get her to take the drugs that I intended for her, I injected them with a very fine needle into the body of the flour worms, which I immediately threw onto the sticky threads of the central trap of the web. In this way I was sure that Héloïse, who completely emptied the worm, also absorbed my mixture. But adroitness was needed, to avoid killing the worm, which had to keep moving right up to the moment when the spider paralysed it prior to digesting it, for any immobile or dead worm was scorned.

When Héloïse had swallowed my poison, she withdrew to the corner of her web. Using a stick with a small scrubbing-brush on the end, I loosened the web in a few seconds, taking care to leave a few remnants at the four principal anchorage points: it was from these points that Héloïse was going to mend her web.

During this reconstruction phase, which often began at night, I positioned myself in a corner of the animal house with an electric torch in my hand, to follow the stages in the making of the web, and to take photographs. I could then assess and measure the effect of drugs on a meticulous, precise, regular and geometrical task, and work out the direction in which deviations in Héloïse's instinctive automatism were operating.

Héloïse did not like mescaline, the alkaloid extract of peyote or peyotl (a hallucinogenic cactus); on the other hand she reacted very well to LSD. The most surprising characteristic of the action of LSD on the spider's web was that, unlike the other hallucinogens, this compound, in small doses, *increased* the regularity of the angles formed between the radial and concentric strands, giving an appearance of greater geometric precision to the web. This seemed paradoxical to me, considering the strong hallucinogenic power of LSD to disturbing sensory input. However, I noticed that Héloïse, under the effect of LSD, worked more regularly, spinning a thinner web without stopping, as if she were following a prepared framework, without taking notice of noises or exterior interference, which would normally distract her, making her stop and then start off again following another angle. Thus, when I lit up the web with my torch to make my nocturnal observations, Héloïse stopped spinning, whereas under LSD she continued her work unperturbed.

Héloïse's webs under LSD allowed me to bring studies of hallucinogens on animal behaviour and movement coordination closer to observations in humans.

Then, one day, Héloïse disappeared. My searches and those of Dupin were in vain, but I kept her last web, which I succeeded in fixing on a piece of tarlatan, for a long time.

In my laboratory I now had a number of techniques to develop models representing mental illness. In creating experimental psychoses in animals, I tried to prepare animals to receive antidote medicines before administering them to humans. Also, I could study the changes that these mind poisons caused in the animal's body. I was not the first to gather together unusual menageries, nor to produce abnormal animals—Henri Baruk had rendered animals catatonic with a substance called bulbocapnine in 1930—but in contrast to those who sought only to study or explain physiopathological, psychopathological or even sociobiological mechanisms, my research had as its chief objective the discovery of drugs that would put right the disorders I had brought about. This research had not escaped the enquiring mind of one illustrious scientist who paid me an unexpected visit one day.

The scientist and the turning mice

One June morning, on arriving at Sainte-Anne, I found sitting on the steps of the little stairway leading to my laboratory, a man in his fifties who was quietly reading a paper. At my arrival he got up, checked who I was, and told me his name which I did not quite catch, but which I hesitated to ask him to repeat. He told me that he worked at the California Institute of

Technology in Pasadena, that he had read my publications about IDPN mice, and that he was hoping to see them. He was in Paris for a symposium on applied wave mechanics organized by Raymond Daudel (in honour of de Broglie), who had given him my address. My visitor was very tall, lean, with a thin head and grey curly hair, spreading onto the temples on either side of a central smooth, shiny bald patch.

I showed him my IDPN mice, which he handled for a while without saying anything. He held them on his hands, on his thighs, and got them to run round on tilting lids. In the end he said to me, 'This is an extraordinary animal.'

He went into an explanation, which I followed with difficulty because it involved smatterings of atomic chemistry tied up with quantum mechanics. It was a question of being able to explain the mechanism of the connection between IDPN and cerebral proteins. According to my visitor, this was the key to a better understanding of the different types of molecular illnesses.

While he was speaking, the telephone rang. It was Raymond Daudel, warning me that I was about to receive a visit from Linus Pauling, the American scientist who had that year received the Nobel prize for chemistry. I answered that he had already been here for an hour.

Linus Pauling, at the end of his remarks, told me that I should go and work with him, and that he would organize a laboratory for me at Pasadena. He offered me an assistant professorship. This did not interest me, because I knew he was only pursuing structure and mechanical research. When, in politely declining, I told him that anybody could produce IDPN mice, and that with his collaborators he could easily study the brain biochemistry of these little creatures without me, he replied, 'He who has discovered something always has a ten-year start on those who repeat the experiment.'

Linus Pauling was a man who was interested in everything. I had an unusual day with him. We left Sainte-Anne on foot, talking all the time. We had lunch at the *Cercle Interallie*, where our walk took us, without being aware of how time was passing. Towards the end of the afternoon, I accompanied him back to his hotel. All this time people had been trying to find him, both at the de Broglie symposium and at the American Embassy.

I have never seen Linus Pauling again. Three months after his visit, I received forms from the California Institute of Technology to make a claim for a bursary at Pasadena. He had put a visiting card in with the papers, on which was written, 'Why not?'. I declined, in polite terms.

Not enough animal trials

From studying abnormal (killer rats) or neurotic animals and from the action of hallucinogenic substances on normal animals, we had found a way of making animal experimental psychosis models. However, the observations were very tricky to interpret. In the case of the hallucinogens, heavy doses had to be used, with no possible comparison with those in humans. Further, the results were often paradoxical, as was the case with the spiders who spun their webs better under hallucinogens. I had also tried LSD on cockroaches to see if intoxication with this substance would modify the structure of the ootheca, the chitinous case with compartments in which the orthopteran's eggs are enclosed. In truth, all this Barnum Circus animal parade would only be useful *a posteriori*, after the major psychotropic drugs had been discovered.

For the time being, a little disappointed with our menagerie, we went back to studying experimental psychoses in humans.

Fabricating human mental illness: 'mind poisons'

Replacing a human being with an animal! This is a travesty, a politically correct farce to try things out, do experiments, and 'see what happens'. But there is no 'mental phenomenon' in animals, and literally speaking no mental diseases—only disorders of behaviour. To discover from within where mental illness starts up, in a head in a whirl, we have to go back to humans themselves.

To set up an experimental psychosis in a volunteer under medical control entails virtually no risk; a hallucinogen being *a priori* 'a natural or synthetic drug which in small or medium doses provokes *reversible* psychiatric syndromes in man' [Jean Delay]. So why not try these powders and elixirs that produce intoxication, and even more, hallucination and delirium?

The attraction of mind poisons

Humans have always been interested in mind poisons such as the hallucinogenic drugs. Why? To meet what need, recognized or unconscious?

People have always sought an artificial paradise to escape from appalling living conditions, relieve physical and mental pain, communicate with the gods, perform sacrificial rites, or simply shake off and drive away boredom. There is also a more general, more universal motivation in this quest, and this is the search for ecstasy, enthusiasm, euphoria and rapture that fires the human engine. At their height, passions often bring the exhilaration of anger, combat, victory, power, sex, artistic creativity or love. Some privileged people find these sources of exhilaration within themselves; many do not, and are condemned to find them in drugs or at the bottom of a glass of alcohol. Artificial and less noble ecstasies—but for a short while effective in dispelling boredom and carrying body and mind off on an adventure.

If these intoxications, these deliriums brought about by hallucinogens or other drugs have attracted sad souls looking for exhilaration that they either do not wish or are unable to find in their lives, some brighter spirits, poets and philosophers, have also sought to draw renewal of their aesthetic visions from them. As for psychiatrists in modern times, they have been interested in them for several reasons. First, the psychological changes brought about by hallucinogens provide models of temporary psychoses whose stages can be studied and analysed. Further, the fact that a chemical product can bring about mental disorders leads one to suppose that some spontaneously developing psychoses may be provoked by biochemical disturbances in our secretions (blood, internal environment, hormones and chemical mediators). Finally, these hallucinogens provide the hope, in looking for antagonists to their actions, of finding new remedies for mental illnesses.

The studies involving bringing about human experimental psychoses also find their scientific justification in a better understanding of the chemical structure of cerebral poisons, of their biochemical mode of action, and of their effect on cerebral metabolism.

However, the poisons, and especially the subjects, have to be chosen.

The choice of poisons

There are many mind poisons. Louis Lewin, the famous Berlin pharmacologist, classified them over sixty years ago. When a new substance is extracted from a plant or synthesized by a chemist, it immediately has its place in one of the groups of Lewin's classification.

And so to produce an experimental psychosis, we do not use *euphorics*, including opium and its derivatives morphine, heroin and codeine, nor cocaine, nor the synthetic analogues of these products. Nor do we use the *intoxicants*: alcohol, ether, chloroform or volatile oils. Still less the *excitants* like betel, kat, caffeine, nicotine and even amphetamines. And *hypnotics* not at all. What we use are the fantasy drugs that alone, and in small doses, give rise to sensory illusions.

The Phantastica

Lewin's *Phantastica*: this term has always seduced me by its evocative power of a walk into the bizarre, adventure in the extravagance of a dream; but several other names have been given to these drugs: *psychedelics*, *psychomimetics* and *psychopathogens*. Jean Delay in his concern for accuracy did not hesitate to construct the neologism '*psychodysleptic*'—not very practical to use, but which etymologically takes full account of these products that 'take over the mind by changing the course of thought'. These are substances 'which disturb mental activity and engender a delirious deviation of judgement, with distortion of appreciation of the values of reality. These drugs generate dreamlike states, hallucinations, and states of confusion or depersonalization.'

More simply, I will call them hallucinogens, without giving up Lewin's term completely.

Besides the hallucinogens of vegetable origin like mescaline (extract of peyote), the cannabinols (hashish and marijuana) and psilocybin (derived from mushrooms), modern chemistry has provided many synthetic hallucinogens such as LSD, and ditran, phencyclidine (Sernylan), and tryptamine or amphetamine derivatives such as STP.

Only a few of these substances are sufficiently well known and studied to permit valid experiments. I will only speak of the most important hallucinogens, whose story ought to be known.

Hashish

It is not well enough known that doctors of the past spoke like everyone else, and wrote memoirs about their work that everybody could understand. This is why I recommend reading the remarkable study by Dr Jacques-Joseph Moreau, physician at the Bicêtre and Salpêtrière, entitled *Hashish and Mental Derangement*, published by De Martin & Masson in Paris in 1845.

Better known under the name of Moreau de Tours, this psychiatrist was the first to study on himself, then on patients, and also on healthy adults, the effects of hashish on the mind. Because of the precision of his description and the scientific analysis of what he observed, his comparisons between dreams and mental illness, and his investigative procedures on animals and humans, Moreau de Tours is incontestably the great forerunner of modern psychopharmacologists.

'I want to pursue medicinal treatment of mental illness,' he said. 'This is purely and simply a nervous disorder and to combat and cure it, there is no need to look anywhere but in ordinary medicine for the weapons we need.' He added, 'I am persuaded that through hashish we should be able to get back to the hidden source of these disorders, so numerous, so varied and so strange, which are included under the collective name of mental illness.'

Let him speak again about hashish:

'By its mode of action on mental faculties hashish gives him who has submitted himself to its strange influence the power of studying on himself the mental disorders which characterize madness, or at least the principal intellectual changes which are the starting point of all the forms of mental derangement.'

To 'convince readers who will have some doubts on these observations,' he added,

'I simply tell what I have observed on myself; I say this with assurance and the certainty of not being mistaken, but I understand your doubts ... I can only give you one piece of advice and you will be convinced if you follow it: do as I did, take hashish, experiment on yourselves, see for yourselves.' Persuaded by the extraordinary action of 'this product so widely spread in oriental countries and almost unknown in Europe, I remain astonished that nobody has taken advantage of it for therapeutics.'

In 1841 Moreau de Tours forced three pigeons and two rabbits to swallow 'very strong doses of pure extract, without any effects other than a little excitation followed by a noticeable drowsiness of short duration.' Regretting not being able to 'repeat these experiments on animals higher up in the scale, such as the cat, dog, and above all, monkeys', he decided to progress from the psychological investigation using small doses, to therapeutic trials.

'I saw there a way of effectively combating the fixed ideas of melancholy patients, breaking the chain of these ideas ... of reawakening the *dozing* intelligence of *stuporous* mentally ill people, or again, to give a little motivation to the spirit of demented patients.'

And he went on to do this.

'I had hashish taken in the form of dawamex (a sweetened and scented electuary paste) in increasing doses (30 grams) immediately after a cup of strong coffee. I gave this to demented, melancholic, and one stuporous mentally ill patient.'

Moreau de Tours objectively reported the effects produced:

'With the demented patients the results (I am only speaking of the therapeutic action here) were almost nil. It was the same for the stuporous patient. The two melancholic patients experienced lively excitement with all the features of cheerfulness and chattering ... Such as it was, the excitement passed, and one, then the other, soon fell back into their former state.'

But Moreau de Tours did not give up.

'It is not certain from such limited results that one can judge the action of any medication. Only having a small amount of hashish I had to be miserly. I could not know if, by trying more often, success would have come, and whether in breaking up their reveries from time to time, the chain of their thoughts would not have come to be broken.'

So what we were going to do, Moreau de Tours had attempted with hashish more than a hundred years earlier.

Hashish is not easy to use; active but toxic derivatives (cannabinols) are extracted from the leaves and flowers of the plant. Other preparations have to be given in large amounts, for the quality of marijuana depends very much on the geographical origin of the product—plants growing in temperate zones are less active than those in India, Syria, Turkey and other countries closer to the tropics. Furthermore, Indian hemp is unstable and little by little loses its activity on exposure to the air.

For all these reasons, experimental psychosis investigations have used mescaline, LSD and psilocybin.

Peyote: the plant that fills the eyes with wonder

The tribes of pre-Columbian America used drugs widely in their religious ceremonies. The Inca priests offered coca leaves to the Sun God; they ate them, probably to have prophetic visions; and the Mexicans used a drug extracted from the sacred mushroom (teonanácatl) and especially peyote.

Louis Lewin talked a lot about peyote, but we are indebted to Alexandre Rouhier for a remarkable study of this little hallucinogenic cactus. It is Rouhier who, in 1927, was to call peyote 'the plant which makes the eyes fill with wonder'. Nearer to our times, the ethnologist Marius Benzi has on several occasions been to live amongst the Huichol Indians, the last ritual users of peyote.

We owe one of the first descriptions of peyote to Father Bernardino de Sahagún, who chronicled the conquest of Mexico by Hernando Cortés:

'The Théochichimecs knew about the grasses and roots, their properties and effects. They were also acquainted with peyote. The peyote eaters consumed it instead of wine. They gathered somewhere on the plain. There, they sang all night and all day. The next day they gathered again and wept a great deal. With their tears, they said, they washed their eyes and purified them. This was when they ate peyote. This is a plant as big as a nopal [cactus], with a white fluffy pappus, which grows in northern regions, and those who eat or drink it have frightening or laughable visions. The intoxication lasts for two or three days, then disappears. The Chichimecs consume a considerable amount of this plant. It gives them strength, excites them for battle, relieves fear, and stops them being affected by hunger or thirst. It is even said that it protects them from all danger.'

The Texan merchants who traded in it at the beginning of the twentieth century bought slices of sun-dried peyote from Mexican traffickers, which they called 'dry whisky' or 'mescal buttons'. The extraction of the active principles of peyote, particularly the active alkaloid mescaline,* renewed interest in the experimental study of this product in humans.

Isolated and identified by the German Arthur Heffter in 1896, mescaline was synthesized by Ernst Späth in 1919. One of the investigators who studied mescaline in humans was K. Beringer, who, with Willy Mayer-Gross, gave a detailed description of the hallucinations induced by the drug. Henri Ey in France was also one of the pioneers of this kind of study.

When I joined Delay at Sainte-Anne, he had already carried out (in collaboration with H. P. Gérard) a number of experiments with mescaline on normal subjects and on psychiatric patients. What interested me was the possibility of getting rid of the mescaline hallucinations with other substances; an antidote for mescaline would perhaps work on the hallucinations of some psychoses. At any rate, study of the chemical relations between the antidote and mescaline was the basis of interesting research.

Well before neuroleptics and tranquillizers—which proved to be powerful antagonists of mescaline—had been discovered, only two substances were effective in reducing the 'mescaline experience': barbiturates and sodium succinate. Intravenous injection of amylobarbitone (a hypnotic) abolished the hallucinations before the onset of sleep. Of more interest was the action of sodium succinate, since this product had practically no true pharmacodynamic action of its own. It only worked through a biochemical pathway. Gérard had asked me to make up some ampoules, and we were able to repeat Schueler's experiments, clearing away hallucinations within a few minutes with three grams of sodium succinate. From that point, trying the experiment on a hallucinatory psychosis only needed a subject to be found.

One day, Gérard announced to me that he had an ideal patient for the experiment: auditory hallucinations set off by the ringing of bells or chimes of clocks. This was a laundress from the Roquette area who one day had an argument with her colleagues, whom she accused of grossly insulting her. This usually happened at midday, when the bell ringing announced the lunch break.

'At the beginning, I thought someone had plugged earphones into the electric irons,' she said. 'When I put the iron near my cheek to feel the warmth, I heard rude remarks.'

At the hospital the patient also heard insulting voices when bells rang or clocks struck. Shaking a bunch of keys near her ears was also enough. I prepared about ten ampoules of sodium succinate, and one

---

* The 'mescal buttons' of peyote must not be confused with Mezcal, a common Mexican alcoholic drink, which is a fermented extract of an agave plant commonly called by the same name.

morning, we proceeded with the experiment. The patient had been shown to Gérard's consulting room. We questioned her. She still heard insults.

'These blasted bitches will have my skin. Here, you can hear it perfectly well, you too!'

We answered evasively, 'Perhaps, but not very well. Not distinctly. All the same, we'll give you an injection which is going to make things better.'

We injected five ampoules. After each, we asked, 'Now, can you still hear it?'

The patient pricked up her ears and gave a very affirmative 'Yes'.

Disappointed, we were going to give up the experiment when I suggested:

'Why not give her some mescaline now?'

We injected 0.40 gram of mescaline sulphate intravenously. After ten minutes the patient hummed, 'Happy days are here again.' She pointed to the wall, 'You see, they're going away, but they say they'll be coming back.'

During the whole day she heard nothing more, but was seized with anxiety which subsided to be replaced by coloured visions, which she described poorly (mostly as a result of lack of culture and vocabulary), but which she strongly resented. On several occasions we asked her if she heard her insulting voices.

'No. That's finished. No more, they have shut their gobs.'

We tried sodium succinate again. The hallucinations faded in a quarter of an hour. We waited anxiously, 'And the voices, the insults?'

She heard nothing more. This lasted the next day, and through the following days. Gérard was delighted; I began to build up superb theories about the oxidation of mescaline involving different substrates. And then on the fourth day, at the moment when a test of sirens was being made in the Glacière area, the old refrain started up again. Everything returned, with the insults and concertos of laundress's cries of rage.

Thousands of observations on mescaline-induced experimental psychoses have been published. I saw Willy Mayer-Gross in Birmingham in 1955, a few years before his death. I had been invited to the Institute of Experimental Psychiatry, which Joel Elkes and Philip Bradley directed, for a conference on the action of hallucinogens on normal and abnormal animals. In the evening, Mayer-Gross invited us to his cottage near the Uffculme Clinic, which, as Senior Fellow, he directed. That evening he recalled the stages of his career at the Heidelberg Clinic, at Groningen, and at the Maudsley Hospital in London. He told us that amongst his numerous investigations, his studies with Beringer on mescaline had given him as much hope as disappointment.

'Mescaline,' he told me, 'is like a box of pastels in the hands of an artist or those of a dauber. The handicapped person remains unresponsive, dumb and blind, whilst a Huxley makes a lyrical portrait with it.'

Herman C. B. Denber and Paul Hoch in New York said almost the same thing to me. When they gave mescaline to schizophrenic patients, they observed an aggravation of symptoms and an even greater psychic disorganization. They were simply stirring the witches' cauldron.

However, I could not stop thinking that less than half a gram of mescaline could render the finest well-balanced heads temporarily delirious. There was a magic in this powder that should have explained many things. Now, all this was only of moderate interest compared with the discovery of LSD, which raised one of the most fascinating problems in modern psychiatry, and unlocked theories on the biochemical origin of certain psychoses.

The adventure in a grain of madness

You weigh out a gram of powdered sugar, which you spread on a visiting card; with a magnifying glass you see the tiny crystals of sugar, and with the point of a needle you pick one out. This sugar crystal weighs about a milligram. Now, suppose you could divide it into ten even smaller fragments; you would only have a few grains of sugar dust, which a puff of breath, would disperse. But if these tenths of a grain are not sugar nor dust but lysergic acid diethylamide, a single one of them placed on your tongue would, in a few moments, empty your head of the daylight and notion of space and replace your normal reason with fantasy or anguish, euphoria, and a distorted view of the world. You have lost your judgement, your willpower, and above all your liberty; and in this sense you will be no different from the herd of people who have to be locked up and confined in asylums.

What gives LSD its incomparable interest is that its extraordinary power of dissolving thought, and depersonalizing the individual, happens with a minute quantity of the substance. Indeed, the storm set off by LSD is as astonishing as a tidal wave started by a seagull's wing would be.

Imagine this grain of LSD, invisible to the naked eye, which you have put on your tongue: it is already taken up by your saliva and dispersed by it into millions of droplets which can linger on the papillae of your tongue and in the tonsillar crypts, but are eventually swallowed into the stomach. There its concentration becomes infinitesimal, these are grains of sand in the ocean; they make their way along the twists and turns of the digestive tract, where, here and there, a few molecules are absorbed, becoming further diluted in our five litres of blood and seventy kilos of flesh. Of these millionths of a grain, what do our brain cells absorb? There lies the mystery and fascination of this drug, which must be placed among the ten great discoveries of the twentieth century, owing to its importance in medical research on the brain. For this action of LSD cannot be a mass action, but a different effect brought about by the triggering of an uninterrupted series of biochemical reactions on the nerve structure receptors—the millions of mini-radar dishes on the millions of cells that made up our kilo of brain substance.

Does this action of LSD, so powerful in minute doses, not open the way to a biochemical concept of the cause of psychoses? Why should not mental illness—real mental illness (so much the worse for those who are going to wince)—be provoked, in psychologically predisposed individuals, by the action of a chemical poison originating in the body itself, and produced in minute quantity and so far not detected by our techniques and apparatus? Certainly, there are too many different mental illnesses for this hypothesis to hold for the thousand disturbances of reason, and particularly for dementia; but the fact remains that after the discovery of LSD scientists have no longer approached mental illness as in the past, with a hood over their head concealing the mechanism from them. They now know that if thought is not entirely inside the brain, in spite of everything one must look there a little when things go off the rails.

LSD or Hofmann's tale

Like many other scientific discoveries, LSD was identified by chance. The circumstances that led to the selection of this product were reported to me by Ernst Rothlin, scientific director of Sandoz, where Albert Hofmann was working, and by the latter himself.

Albert Hofmann is a willingly talkative man, whom I have met several times. In the course of a Society of Therapeutic Chemistry symposium, organized by Pierre Tronche at Clermont-Ferrand, I found myself invited with him to a reception at the château at Chazeron. I got him to taste cherry liqueur mixed with kirsch, a drink he had not met before, and of which he drank several glasses.

'You'll have to lead me back to the hotel!' he jokingly told me.

When I replied that the aperitif was less toxic than LSD, he told me his story in detail.

'It was in 1938 that I prepared LSD for the first time, in the context of a study on the semi-synthetic alkaloids of rye ergot.'

Ergot is produced by a parasitic fungus, *Claviceps purpurea*, which contaminates grains, principally rye. In the Middle Ages, in rainy summers whole harvests of rye were spoiled by this fungus. When the population, out of ignorance, indifference or forced by starvation, ate bread made with such contaminated flour, some people saw their hands and feet become gangrenous. This disease was also called 'St Anthony's fire' or 'Ardents' disease' because the fingers and toes looked as if they had been charred. This flour also caused abortions, visual disturbances, and even mental disorders, in the form of epidemics of mental illness that were thought to be contagious.

Ergot contains a large number of active substances, including ergotamine, a powerful vasoconstrictor that midwives have used since 1836 to arrest haemorrhages in childbirth. The mental illnesses seen in the Middle Ages, caused by ergotism did not arise from a hallucinogenic property of the fungus, but from massive doses of alkaloid vaso-constrictors, and no doubt also from hysterical reactions provoked by the alarming appearance of the gangrenous limbs.

Wanting to obtain a pure preparation of ergot, and to find out about its chemical constituents, the Sandoz laboratories at Basle entrusted this work to the great chemist Arthur Stoll and to his assistant Albert Hof-mann. As a result, Stoll and Hofmann discovered that the fundamental constituent of the ergot alkaloids was an acid with an indole structure, which they called lysergic acid (*Lyserg Säure* in German). As well as this acid, they identified many other ergot alkaloids, of which many were studied by the pharmacologist Rothlin, and recommended in the treat-ment of migraine and sympathetic nervous system disorders. One of the best-known of Sandoz's products, Hydergine, used as a cerebrovascular medication, is a mixture of alkaloid derivatives and lysergic acid deriva-tives.

To make these products, Stoll and Hofmann carried out what is known as a semi-synthesis. From ergot collected from cultures of rye specially contaminated for the purpose, all the alkaloids were extracted and sub-jected to alkaline hydrolysis to obtain lysergic acid from which the other compounds could be synthesized.

'I reckoned,' Hofmann told me, 'on making a cardiotonic compound analogous to Coramine [a Ciba product containing nikethamide], a known circulatory stimulant, and which is the diethylamide of nicotinic acid. So I synthesized the diethylamide of lysergic acid, and as this was the twenty-fifth of a new series, I designated it LSD 25 [Lysergsäure-diäthylamid].'

Just five years later, Hofmann once more synthesized this product, this time at the request of the pharmacologists.

'It was April the sixteenth 1943, and I was overtaken, at the labora-tory, by an odd feeling of dizziness and agitation. Objects, and the appearance of my laboratory workers, seemed to undergo optical changes. I was unable to concentrate on my work. I left the labora-tory as if in a dream, and went home, where I was overcome by an irresistible need to lie down and sleep. The daylight seemed unpleasantly bright. I drew the curtains. I went off to sleep right away in a state of intoxication, associated with wild imagination. With eyes closed, fantastic images, of extraordinary plasticity, and harsh colours as in a kaleidoscope seemed to loom up in front of me. After two hours things gradually settled down and I had a meal, which I enjoyed, feeling back to normal and quite well.'

'I attributed these symptoms to chance intoxication with a very small amount of LSD 25. Having clarified matters, I tried an experiment on myself which turned out badly, for the dose of 0.25 mg which I took, thinking it was very weak, turned out subsequently to be five times more than an average active dose.'

Albert Hofmann had asked one of his co-workers to accompany him home. Because of the petrol restrictions at the time, he was riding a bicycle. To get home, he had to cross a bridge over the Rhine. 'I had to get off my bike and stay sitting on the bridge, unable to move.'

This time, the symptoms lasted much longer and Hofmann was examined by a psychiatrist. Arthur Stoll, director of the chemistry department at Sandoz, and Hofmann's boss, had a son who was assistant to Manfred Bleuler at the Zürich psychiatric clinic. Called by his father to Hofmann's bedside, Willy Stoll took note of the psychiatric disturbances that his father's collaborator presented, and which he went on to report during the years 1948–1950 to several medical societies.

From 1951, Delay and Pichot in France, Mayer-Gross in England, Rinkel in Boston and Hoch in New York repeated the self-observations of Hofmann and Stoll with LSD that the Sandoz laboratories kindly issued to psychiatric centres and research laboratories. The Sandoz company even launched LSD 25 under the trade name Delysid. For a while the product was used in experimental psychiatry studies, to analyse the development of 'psychosis models' in normal subjects and to attempt to clarify the nature, mechanism and structure of certain mental disorders. However, the effect of LSD on various types of patient resulted in its use 'being recommended in the course of psychotherapy, either to change affective relationships or emotional tone favourably, or to promote the revival of emotionally highly charged memories.'

Hundreds of studies were carried out throughout the world, and by 1966 there were more than a thousand articles, papers and progress reports dealing with this extraordinary hallucinogen. The study of experimental mental illness was fuelled by widespread curiosity.

Curiosity may be commendable, but there is also a need for discretion. The great discovery of LSD led to both good and bad results in exciting curious minds. First, there was the curiosity of scientists and of psychiatrists, which might have been profitable and may yet be so one day. Then there was the egotistical curiosity of the intellectuals, which leads on to the morbid and dangerous curiosity of the 'poor souls'.

LSD and scientific curiosity

We have all had wonderful dreams. At one stroke we thought we knew everything. When there is a poison, there is an antidote; the discovery of a virus often precedes a vaccine; microbes and bacteria have their antibiotics. We had mental illness in microcrystals, delirium in homeopathic suspension. An active, calculated dose of a few hundred million

LSD molecules, thrown at our fourteen billion nerve cells, was the detonator that it sufficed to defuse. Surely, the mechanism would be found and dismantled. One day the action of LSD on the neuron was discovered, the next day its action on the barrier between the brain and the meninges, and the following week on nerve transmission. Then there was the succession of sensational communications from John Henry Gaddum, Bernard Brodie and Erminio Costa, David Woolley and David Shaw, and Abram Hoffer and Humphrey Osmond: *LSD is the most powerful serotonin antagonist.* And as serotonin was at that time fashionable (Vittorio Erspamer and Irvine Page had found that this neurotransmitter was essential for normal brain function) it was thought that everything had been demonstrated.

Like so many others, I had made my contribution, with measurements, unpublished tests, and an analysis of the two phases of action of LSD, stimulant then paralysing. We thought that we had the devil by the tail, and were waiting for him to keel over. Sandoz put out the flags. Rothlin first, then Aurelio Cerletti, his assistant, who was to succeed him, started to give worldwide lecture tours. All you had to do was to announce a small discovery of some particular action, and you received some LSD and an invitation to Basle. Hofmann himself started leaving his laboratory and giving lectures.

At the time, in world pharmacology circles, everyone envied the Sandoz scientific team for its great influence. Hofmann's fame was completed by two other spectacular discoveries: the active principle of the famous Aztec hallucinogen teonanácatl, derived from a fungus that Gordon and Valentina Wasson, assisted by Roger Heim, professor of mycology at the Paris Museum, had succeeded in identifying as *Psilocybe mexicana.* He also described and synthesized psilocybin, which Jean Delay was to try subsequently on himself. But Hofmann made yet another sensational discovery: that of the chemical composition of another hallucinogenic substance, the ololiuqui of the Zapotec Indians in the Oaxaca area. He found lysergic acid amide in ololiuqui seeds. When he announced this, botanists and chemists did not want to believe him, because for them lysergic derivatives only existed in the lower fungi. It was thought that he was mistaken: some even said that in his laboratory the LSD which lay around everywhere had contaminated the preparation. When other chemists like Toher and Heacock also found lysergic acid amide in ololiuqui, enthusiasm developed; the connection was made between the most powerful hallucinogen synthesized artificially, and the hallucinogen of the Aztecs: between the modern drug and the old magic drugs.

Of what interest, one may ask, is all this for the mental hospital inmate who walks around or loiters in the asylum courtyard for long days and months?

Science is made from these fertile enthusiasms. Scientists' shouts of joy, puerile perhaps, ring out in the corridors of discovery. LSD and all these experiments were believed in. Men like Aurelio Cerletti, Hofmann and all the scientists I have named gambled their fame and careers, like politicians, hoping to avoid recantations. Apart from all that, there remained nevertheless the remarkable chemical work of Hofmann, and increasingly precise biochemical psychopharmacological techniques. I am sure that it was all praiseworthy and useful.

LSD and psychiatrists' curiosity

If the scientists in their laboratories wanted to understand and find things out, the doctors and the psychiatrists wanted to be adventurous and play with fire. Many took the poison themselves, but they also played with others—volunteers—healthy and sick, and became heavily involved in observing the ordeal of mental illness. These clinicians have seen people become gods or devils, free like heroes or crucified with anguish—but either way brought out of themselves by the drug. The enquiring psychiatrist has studied wisely, using drugs, including LSD, to understand, to provide care, and to facilitate psychotherapy. Remarkable clinical observations, and strange or curious mental disturbances, have come to be analysed. Patients have been helped, and others cured, thanks to experimental psychoses, and to modifications of outlook on the world brought about by the hallucinogens.

I remain persuaded that even if such procedures cannot come into general use outside the hospital setting and under medical supervision, they are still a justifiable and useful approach.

LSD and morbid curiosity

Then there is the herd of other interested people, those who go astray.

First, the herd of well-made heads, or those who claim to be such: intellectuals who want to experiment and join in the game. The dismal adventure of Timothy Leary, in charge of psychology teaching at Harvard, is well known. This academic wanted to study the 'increased awareness' with psychochemistry: the possibility of the mind expanding to embrace and grasp everything. For him, LSD and the other hallucinogens made this possible. They were 'cerebral vitamins' that we lacked, and without which we were deprived of the ability to see the world properly and attain true understanding. No longer a drug, LSD was a nutrient of the mind, and it was natural justice for each of us to have it. The restrictions governing LSD and the legal obligations for its prescription were considered by him an abuse of power and a deliberate restriction to undernourished populations.

Leary, with his colleague Alpert, founded the International Foundation for Internal Freedom (IFIF). They distributed thousands of doses of LSD and psilocybin to Harvard students to do their own experiments.

Driven from the USA, Leary went to Acapulco, where he turned a disused hotel into a boarding-house where he welcomed the students who had followed him, and where, for $200 a month and $6 for a dose, they could drug themselves at will. Driven from Mexico, Leary went back to New York State, where he started the 'Castalia Foundation' near the colleges of Vassar and Bennett. Yoga and meditation were taught there, but mescaline and LSD were also distributed. Hundreds of young people still followed his mystical teaching, which they spread in the colleges, schools and universities of the USA. At last, arrested for a minor offence, Leary was condemned to jail.

As well as these intellectual propagators of dangerous ideologies, there was also another herd of 'poor souls' or acid heads who rush forwards to prove to themselves that they still know how to walk.

Their experience usually begins with an 'acid party', followed by a couple of trips each month, with perhaps a little drink impregnated with LSD, diluted in a glass of water, or a little sugar saturated with a hundred micrograms of the product. Sometimes the young novices who are trying the drug for the first time will have a 'guide', an initiator who will control the experiment; the guide takes a weaker dose to stay lucid and join in the fun, and get into 'contact' with the novices. The guide will explain their visions to the others, soothe their eventual terrors, and help them to 'receive communion with the universe'. In this new world of hallucinations and sensory illusions, the normal scenery of life loses all reality. Often the interactions and communication with the guide are made without words, 'each penetrating the thoughts of the other'.

These experiments are repeated at closer intervals, as the hold of the hallucinogenic adventure becomes stronger. Interest in normal activities fades away, and eventually the person 'drops out', abandoning school, work and home, to sink down into a drug community.

I will not enlarge on what is no more than toxicomania, as it is beyond my subject of experimental psychiatry, but it must be said that LSD has joined the drugs that give rise to addiction. It has created a particular kind of addiction owing to its own actions (I was going to say qualities).

The best and the worst

I was fascinated by the experimental research carried out with LSD in laboratory animals, on the biochemical mechanisms of their antagonisms with the mediators and neurohormones of the brain. At the same time, I also experimented on humans.

The aim was the creation in the patient of a kind of 'deep introspection' leading to a better understanding of self. The doctor and the patient had to choose, from amongst the hallucinations that occurred during the experiment, the most significant and the most apt to facilitate an analysis.

Sometimes another technique was also used: a large dose (more than 200 micrograms, up to half a milligram) was administered to give rise to complete loss of consciousness. A 'death–resurrection', to use Sidney Cohen's expression, was provoked, from which the patient could emerge with a completely changed behaviour.

It is this last technique that my friend Bernard P employed with good results.

I often assisted him at his experiments, which I helped him to control. He obtained remarkable cures in certain cases of neurosis and psychosis, using the phase during which the subject, under the influence of LSD, was in a state of hypersuggestibility. The patient, who relived the dramatic event that had generated the illness, could be freed from it in the course of an emotional discharge, all the more easily since the patient was at that exact moment deprived of all critical spirit and accepted all the doctor suggested as gospel truth.

This was truly the best of LSD: the remodelling of a mind, first destroyed or emptied, washed, then reconstructed and furnished with the kind words of the psychotherapist whom the patient never thought to doubt. Unfortunately, this best could turn to the worst when the 'reawakened dreamer' under LSD escaped from the control of a guide or witness; for the abolition of all critical spirit delivered the subject up to unusual impulses, at the command of a hallucination or brought about by deep-rooted inclinations in the subject's nature and character.

This will be more easily understood after reading the following accounts.

The best of Basambo Daka

He arrived very late at my Monday session, and Madame B, the head nurse, asked me if I could still see him.

'It's half-past twelve, we don't take more appointments after eleven o'clock. I'll tell him to come back tomorrow.'

'What's the matter with him?'

'He's a student from the City university. A negro.'

'We say a Black or an African, Madame B.'

'If you like, but what shall I tell him?'

'I'll see him. There won't be any more for a while.'

As soon as the patient was seated in front of me, he took a handkerchief from his pocket and mopped his face, and at once a heavy, strong perfume invaded the room. He kept the handkerchief, which gave off a penetrating odour, in his hand. I do not know how he saw on my face my dislike of breathing this tenacious stench, for he immediately asked me, 'Doctor, you can smell it too?'

'Smell what?'

'My odour.'

'I can certainly smell the perfume coming from your handkerchief, and perhaps your clothes. It is a very strong perfume.'

'No, doctor—you are not telling me the truth, it's me you can smell. You smell my bad odour. It's me. I am going rotten.'

On this evidence, the consultation was going to be prolonged. Perhaps hospital admission would be needed. I warned the head nurse and started to question my patient.

I will conceal his true name. I will call him Daka, Basambo Daka. He had come from his country of Senegal to study arts in Paris. He lived in the City university and since his arrival in Paris everything had been going well for him. He had even succeeded in getting a small volume of verse accepted by an editor, which he intended to dedicate to Léopold Sédar Senghor. And then, one evening . . .

'I love Sitia, I have loved her for ever. It is true. We are friends, but I want to marry her. She knows this. I knew her in Dakar and we found one another again in Paris. She is a Tukulor with Peul blood and I am a Tukulor with Ouolof blood . . .'

Basambo stopped at times to overcome suppressed emotion which broke into sobs. He wiped his eyes and blew his nose noisily, and his shaken handkerchief again set free very strong smells.

That evening Sitia had said to him, 'Basambo, you must change your perfume.'

I made no remark, but thought how right Sitia was. Undoubtedly, Basambo read my thoughts.

'No, doctor, it was not this perfume. It was a light mixture of citronella and cardamom. I like perfumes a lot, it is my mother who taught me to recognize them. She had a large collection of them in dogwood flasks. What Sitia smelt, doctor, was my bad smell. I am going rotten inside. I am decomposing. That is why I have changed my perfume; now it is a new mixture which my mother has sent me, with neruli and opopanax, and especially musk. It's to hide my smell. Doctor, I smell bad. Something is rotting inside me.'

Basambo had already consulted several doctors, at the Cochin hospital and Hôtel-Dieu; general physicians, ear, nose and throat specialists, and dentists. He had been told there was nothing wrong, and that there was nothing to smell. But he knew himself he was going to die and was already decomposing. He kept away from Sitia and no longer wanted to see her, but she had come back to comfort him. She told him that he was giving himself ideas, that she had only smelt his perfume, and that it was ridiculous to imagine such things.

'She again advised me to change my perfume because she finds it too strong, but in fact, it is my odour which is bothering her.'

Basambo asserted to me that if he removed the perfumes with which he anointed his whole body and spread over his clothes, it would be a catastrophe.

'The whole world would smell the odour of my decaying carcass.'

Everything I could say to Basambo was useless. He wept, perspired, and rubbed his nose and hands with his handkerchief. My consulting room was overcome by his perfume. I longed to open the window to change the air, but I could not do this for fear of increasing his distress even more by being taken wrongly.

'Why have you come to Sainte-Anne? What can I do for you since you do not believe what I say to you?'

It was Sitia who had persuaded him to come to a psychiatric centre for a consultation. She had told him that his stories of decomposition and of rotting were 'bad ideas' and that at Sainte-Anne there were specialist doctors for this, who treated bad ideas.

'I am not mad, doctor. I agreed to come to please her.'

He confessed as well that she had come with him, that she was in the garden in front of the clinic, and that she was waiting for him. With his agreement, I got her to come in. She was a slim girl with a supple gait, dressed in a brown silk wrap, with a shaakri hairstyle and large gold bands. She confirmed everything Basambo Daka had told me, but her comments together with mine had no persuasive effect upon her friend.

I was going to prescribe sedatives and barbiturates, then recommend a further consultation with a psychotherapeutic psychiatrist, when at that very moment my colleague Bernard P came into my consulting room to ask me something. I got up for a moment; in an aside he wondered at the fierce perfume which had overtaken the room, and I told him, in a few sentences, Basambo's story.

'Give him some LSD,' he advised me. 'He will forget all his smells.'

I recognized Bernard P's great experience and his encouraging results. With Sitia's help I got Basambo to agree to giving this a try.

A witchdoctor again

We asked him to come without perfume, but he didn't listen to us.

'I've just used some lavender.'

He swallowed a glass of water and seemed surprised.

'You haven't given me a pill.'

We explained to him that the medication was in the glass, but in such a small quantity that the taste was imperceptible.

He started to 'take off', he told us, forty-five minutes later. I will summarize the five hours which the procedure, organized and conducted by Bernard P, occupied.

Basambo was drifting in scenes of sound and colours; only 'images' of his odours remained, without any affective tone, pleasing or painful; but the 'wonder' for him came from a return to his native Africa. He relived his childhood. Eldest son of a village chief, cherished by an attentive mother, educated at the college in Dakar and for each holiday period a return to the bush, tribal life, thatched huts, wells, herds of goats, which he loved taking to the backwater. Trips to the market town of N'Mambé where Sitia lived. Then one day the big departure to France. The farewells to father and mother in the chief's hut.

'Basambo, I give you my blessing. But you must do something for me.'

'Yes, mother.'

'Go and see M'Umba, the witchdoctor, and ask him for a charm to protect you while you are in France.'

Basambo tried to make his mother understand that this was all super-stition, which was no longer acceptable—outdated fetishism. But mother Daka looked so sad seeing her son leave that he promised to go and see M'Umba in his hut at the edge of the village, behind the hedge of prickly bushes that protected his straw hut.

He sat down in front of the witchdoctor, explained what his mother wanted, and M'Umba had the satisfaction of seeing Basambo, who since his long stays in Dakar had disdained his services and denigrated him amongst the village men, come back. The witchdoctor selected a small bag of hare-skin hanging from a cord, and put a jackal's tooth, a harrier's claw and a few feather barbs into it. He chanted a few words.

'There, Basambo, here is your charm for the journey. But you tell your father he must give me a goat.'

Basambo was appalled by this exorbitant barter, and the imposition of the witchdoctor on his mother's credulity. He threw the charm in M'Umba's face and injured him. So M'Umba was very angry. He threat-ened him, and threw a curse at the religious renegade.

'You will rot amongst the Whites who have already contaminated you. I, M'Umba, tell you. With them you will become like an ox carcass. You will be carrion for the white vultures.'

All this Basambo now recalled, in the middle of this fantastic voyage that he made deep into himself under the power of LSD.

Basambo is split apart, divided into a hundred characters. He is at once the witchdoctor and the old chief; he is also his mother and Sitia; he plays his roles, as he plays feast scenes and childhood fantasies, his life in the wild, holidays in his village, his encounters with the witchdoctor of whom he was always afraid as a child, and made fun of later on.

'It's him, M'Umba who has bewitched me; who has cast a spell on me, and put a curse on me and is making me rot away.'

Basambo got up from the bed on which he was lying; he stared at the wall and drew an imaginary figure with his finger. Now he speaks a dialect we do not understand, very quickly, with menacing gestures.

'Basambo, it's all done. What can you see now? What can you hear?'

We took Basambo back to an armchair near a table where there was an apparatus recording what he said. There was now calmness and peace on Basambo's face. He asked us what to write about, but remained motionless in front of the blank page. We gave him a light cold meal, for the procedure was taking a long time. He ate and drank slowly. The he asked to go to the toilet. On returning, he pounced upon his sheet of paper and began to write.

'Liquorice juice and little nipper,
   Liquorice juice and little nipper'

— this repeated more than twenty times. And under the last line,

   'Bébe coal has sold us'

— and he signed his page of writing, which he held out to us with satisfaction.

We asked him about what he had seen and heard and about the smells he noticed. He shook his head, smiling, in a relaxed and happy manner. After a moment he said, 'Certainly I no longer smell anything.'

He told us later that at first he had been frightened of the procedure to which he was going to be submitted, and that he suddenly felt happy because he saw the light of the sun through the window. The sun made him more happy than anything else in the world; it lit up the things around him and these objects were wonderful: the table, the bed, a book resting on the bed. Suddenly everything seemed unreal to him; the wall half-opened, and he was in his native village, living through a day in his childhood. His mother, his father and the witchdoctor M'Umba were there, who each in turn repeated to him, jokingly, what he had told Bernard P and me with much distress and anger. There was a considerable difference between the good humour and overflowing joy which Basambo had lived through in his procedure and the dramatic spectacle with which we had seen him involved.

'The sandwich you gave me, and the glass of water with it, were for me the most extraordinary meal I have ever had,' he told us. When we had shown him what he had written, he told us, very disappointedly, that he had believed he was composing the most beautiful poem in the world.

Basambo now clearly remembered the witchdoctor's curse and could understand his olfactory hallucinations.

Bernard P gave him two more LSD sessions, which I did not attend. One day he called me to introduce me to the cured Basambo. I was happy about this fine result, but for some time it had been my friend who was worrying me.

The best for the worst

My conversations with Bernard P came to a sudden end when we talked about our work. We countered or backed up our opinions on many subjects with arguments that we defended according to our temperaments, but there was never any convergence regarding our medical vocation.

'By wanting to look after mental illness, you are despising it,' he told me.

I could not accept this, and he shrugged his shoulders at my fierce replies about the doctor's obligation to treat, and if possible, to cure.

'So much the better for you, if you enjoy it.'

I reproached him for his pessimism over the progression of illness, and also for the distaste for living that he displayed too often. He answered:

'I have been vaccinated against sorrow and boredom, and my mental fatigue is a habit. I chose psychiatry to compare myself with others.' He added, 'And besides, I too believe in therapeutics.'

When the use of hallucinogens began, he quickly became interested in clinical experiments and was one of the first to codify the technique. I remember his visit to my laboratory. He wanted to know everything about LSD, our animal trials, the history of the product, and how its action was explained. It was the first time I had found him so interested in anything.

'I tried the product on my little florist, and it was extraordinary.'

He had already spoken to me about this young girl admitted for an anxiety neurosis with phobia after a rape attempt.

'If you'd seen the kid. An hour after having taken the LSD she was transformed. She started repeating "I am a ladybird. I am a ladybird," and she studied a wisp of black wool in the hollow of her hand. Then she got on her bed and said "Now, it doesn't matter." This morning she told me some extraordinary things. She was immensely happy during the whole experiment. She visited a wonderful countryside where everything was fine, harmonious and reassuring. She was in the air and on the ground at the same time. She remembered the detail of the wisp of wool in her hand—"I could see perfectly well that this was a thread of wool," she told me, 'but I wanted it to be a ladybird".'

Bernard P talked to me for a long time that day. He was surprised and intrigued. He had already planned for two other patients to act as experimental controls. Some time afterwards, he came to explain his trials with LSD on student volunteers to me.

'The same thing happened each time. Three-quarters of an hour after swallowing the dose, they took off. They walked on water. They were no longer afraid of anything. They understood things from the inside. They said that the colour perceived is an ocean where they went to drown, drinking the colour; sound satisfies them with beauty, and if you speak of death to them, they hold out their hand towards its spectre as one welcomes a friend.'

He pointed his forefinger to his chest.

'And it is me—we—who set this off with a few pinches of powder. We are great wizards. I assure you: some patients take me for a great wizard and I get very good results by influencing them through suggestion in the right direction.' He continued, 'Tomorrow, can you give up your afternoon for me? I want to try LSD on myself. I would like you to assist me during the event.'

Unsuccessfully, I tried to dissuade Bernard. I was still suspicious about the toxicity of LSD, not because of what I had seen in animals, who tolerated doses that were relatively considerable in comparison with the minimal amounts given to humans, but because of the strangeness of the discordant reactions in volunteers or patients, which gave the doctor the impression of a disturbing disorganization of the personality, whereas the subject recounted his real-life experience as a moment of supreme happiness. At any rate, I did not think that taking LSD was a good thing for Bernard P, too inclined to use and even abuse alcohol and stimulants to dispel a psychasthenic tendency.

He did not give in to my reasoning, but I nevertheless attended him during the six hours that the session lasted. He only took fifty micrograms of LSD, but the reaction he showed impressed me very much, for it was more like that of the patients than that of the theoretically normal volunteers.

After taking the product, he progressively sank into a state of prostration from which I drew him with difficulty to make him say a few words. At one moment, he slowly got up from the armchair where he was sitting, walked about in the room, and abruptly, violently, punched the wall with his fist, then came back to sit down, prostrate once more. A psychiatrist not informed of the experiment would not have been able to distinguish my friend's attitude from that of a schizophrenic patient in a ward. The psychological tests we had agreed to put him through also testified to mental disturbance in the direction of regression towards psychosis and automatism (a schizophrenic state). We had set up a tape recorder to record what he said, but when I questioned him his replies were irrelevant. At one point he lifted his hand as if to get my attention, and hummed the first bars of Mozart's *Turkish March*, but he quickly stopped and resumed his immobile bearing.

When he appeared to me to have resumed normal behaviour and thought processes, I accompanied him to his home. During the drive, he pointed out all the crossing traffic lights.

'Watch the red light.'

'I can see it perfectly well,' I answered, irritated.

At his home a supper had been prepared, which we ate together. I tried to question him again, but he contented himself with saying:

'It's fine. It's all right. It's difficult to express. I'll explain it to you tomorrow.'

The next day I discovered in Bernard P a completely different character. He was cheerful, voluble, and his face expressed a satisfaction I had never caught in him before.

'You must understand, you must understand me. I have had an unforgettable experience, although everything had appeared natural and true to me. I saw you but I forgot your presence. Time only existed for me to take it in bits, to wrap up the events which loomed up. Each time you questioned me, it was almost a form of torture, for you were tearing me away from an infantile happiness which I was sharing with colours, sounds, and objects of which I perceived the least details as achievements and masterpieces. The old penholder which has been on my desk for months was more beautiful than Michelangelo's *Muse*, and the furniture of the room was more sumptuous than the royal apartments at Versailles.'

'At one point, irritated by your questions which loomed as obstacles to my happiness, I got up to get rid of an intruder and I struck the wall violently. I felt severe pain, but curiously, extraneous to me, as if it had stayed on the wall, to harm the wall, but my fist was not painful; on the contrary even, if it were possible, my fist was happy, relieved of its pain. I knew I was keeping still, and I wondered if you were surprised by this, but I could not detach myself from the beauty of everything around me.'

'When you made me take some tests, I would have cursed you, but I tried hard to answer properly, for I did not want to let myself be dragged off by what I thought to be my lapse of memory and the fear of appearing to be a stranger to myself, tasting a happiness which astonished me by its immensity. At one moment my body appeared to be so light that my head seemed detached from it until a wall of sound, and music appeared, which I passed through: this happened when you started up the tape recorder. Setting off the apparatus set free a flood of music, in the middle of which I floated. I walked on the sounds, on the notes, and incorporated myself into the melody; followed it, played it, and sang it without understanding it. I wondered why I was so free, why everything was so good, whereas everything seemed so simple, so normal.'

Bernard P was inexhaustible, and I could not stop wondering at the contrast between the richness of his memories and his constrained attitude and mutism during the experiment.

'When you took me back home, you grumbled about the red lights. I was surprised, because for me it was not any longer a barrier, a prohibition, but a silken colour, of dazzling beauty, which, with the sounds made up a garland. Yes, it was indescribable, but I saw a garland of lights and sounds.'

Bernard stopped for a moment. 'When I sensed that the effect of the LSD was beginning to wear off, I was so sad and depressed at losing such happiness that I thought the deprivation of such joy would lead to my death. Shall I tell you that I have seen it—death? It is perhaps not certain but something came to me which was death, and which explained to me that death was not the absurd end of life, but that it had its place in man's adventure, in man's exploration.'

Bernard P continued like this for a long time, while I wrote down what he said. I had never seen him so happy, drunk with happiness. But his joy left little room for what I had hoped to find within him: the calmness and peace of mind, and the serenity that he told me he had found in the drug but which had gone away as the drug wore off, and which he sought in life in vain. On the contrary, from then on it became Bernard's incessant quest to zero in anew on the border of this impossible universe that he had visited as a dazzled traveller. He repeated the LSD sessions with volunteers and also with patients, but apart from the analyses and interesting results that he drew from his experiments, he found in neither the attitude nor the behaviour of his subjects any reflection of the rapture that had filled him. It is only their accounts, often imperfectly reported, that stirred him the most, because he found in them echoes of his own experience and a reminder of that strange beauty he had experienced. The pressing desire to resume taking the drug himself became more and more insistent, and he had another session, then another. I only learnt this later on, when I expressed surprise that he no longer complained about the lack of talent in his patients for describing their hallucinations.

'I help them with my own experiments,' he told me, and he confessed to me that he had taken LSD, again several times. He did this at home, without medical supervision or any control. He just warned his servant to wake him up the next morning if he was still sleeping after eight hours.

Nothing I said to him had any effect. We quarrelled when one day he asked me for some LSD, which I refused. I was not a drug distributor for clinical trials, but I had a large supply for my laboratory experiments. I sometimes helped out clinicians who were waiting to receive some from Sandoz.

My disagreement with Bernard did not last long; he came back to see me and tried to convince me of the interest of his experiments.

'I will give you a faithful account of my observations, and you will surely draw interesting conclusions from this for your research.'

Knowing the uselessness of all my efforts at dissuasion, I shrugged my shoulders and told him he was playing with fire.

I wish I could say I was wrong. And to this tale, whose only value lies in the facts it report, I wish I could add that there was nothing useless or tragic about experiments by psychiatric doctors with LSD. But Bernard P committed suicide, and whatever effect his underlying mental state had on this act, it is certain that LSD had an influence in this drama, and that it precipitated it.

In the summer following his first experiments, Bernard P left for the Balearic Islands; after staying on Mallorca and Ibiza, he rented a fisherman's house on Formentera where he isolated himself for several weeks with a friend who had gone with him, and who told me what happened.

On the beach at Espalma d'Or every night Bernard joined up with a drug community. There each night a feast took place whose delirious stages were passed through one by one. In groups, they got in the sea and knelt in the waves until they were submerged; silent or screaming, happy or terrified, they communed in a total trance, in utter bliss. Some drowned themselves in the bay. For Bernard, it was a fall from the cliff top where the lighthouse stands, with a precipitous drop down to the sea. A letter was passed on to me, addressed to me: 'At Berheria, I will climb the wild coastal path, and there I will once more be in that harmonious and reassuring world . . .' Everything in this letter was paradoxically treated with calmness and reason, and the discordance with the drama and tragedy was striking, as it was in Bernard's account of his experiments, preserved on the tape recorder.

Bernard's suicide upset me considerably. I had for several years found in my laboratory research, strictly associated with observations on patients, a strong motivation to pursue my psychiatric career, in the hope of one day participating in the initiation of new and rational therapies. Making models of psychoses and studying them proved to be very useful—even necessary—but it was dangerous. This risk of provoking conflicts and dramas was not what I wanted or looked for in my work. Too strange, too tragic in its intent and finality, experience with LSD should not be turned into a rout. I wanted to see, to understand, and perhaps establish a possible reason for all this.

A unique experiment

In the course of my career as doctor, psychiatrist and pharmacologist, I have had prepared (and prepared myself) and studied many drugs and medicines, but I have only rarely taken any, and only if my body felt the need. So I must confess to the fears and apprehensions that I had before taking any LSD. Nevertheless, I wanted to try this drug that could send your mind beyond reason, change your view of the world, modify colour and the duration of time, and embellish the image of death to the point of making it desirable. Then, on an exceptional occasion, I also saw, heard, and felt living 'outside me', the individual who I am.

'These images, sounds, details, colours which appear, get fatter, magnified, disproportionate, dazzling, I feel them, admire them, they gratify me and scare me. Like a tourist who visits a monument, a beauty spot, a museum, I searched the innermost recesses of my mind for this spirit which I feel ten times, a hundred times, lost and found again. I am not talking nonsense, I am examining everything from outside. I have lost my reason. Suddenly I have felt a state of hyperawareness, as it may have loomed up in the soul of the prophets and mystics. My perceptions are identifiable as object, at the same time as the border which separates me from the outside world fades. I am just as much behind my pen as with it and in it, and my carcass no longer weighs its body weight, so that I think I can move myself without touching the ground which is elastic, soft and smooth like a thick carpet.'

'Freed from reality, aiming for a hazy goal which I believe is logical, with all critical sense lost, I plunge into a world where I think and feel with mental images and dreams. My reason has given way to reveries—to dreams. My identity becomes confused with the world, and my perceptions, foreign to the usual manner of their conventions, set free strange, bizarre, and illogical poetic thoughts . . .'

I wrote these sentences after taking LSD, a few hours after returning to what I thought to be a normal mental state. I had been worried for several hours, but never frightened; I had lucid intervals, then again phases of mental fuzziness, and this went on for half a day. Three days after the experiment, one morning at about eleven o'clock, I abruptly experienced turmoils analogous to those I felt during the trial, but this lasted less than a minute. It was as if a few traces of LSD, stuck in a deep recess of my body, perhaps in my brain, had been set free belatedly to produce this effect, in the same way that fireworks, badly fused by the manufacturer, go off after the final climax of the display.

This trial was essential for me, to understand not only the interest but also the dangers of this drug.

The hallucinogenic experience with LSD had revealed to me the existence of exceptional mental states; it helped me to understand what 'disintegration' of the consciousness in the psychoses can represent. I also grasped what 'integration' of sensory phenomena during visionary states and moments of ecstasy in mystics and prophets could be. But, unlike prophets and mystics, I did not retain the conviction of having met the truth, after the LSD trial. This experience remained, in spite of a certain helpful memory, a meagre miracle of the juxtaposition of strange happiness and disturbing anguish.

Unlike Bernard P and all those who hoped to continue their quest for escapism using LSD, I was not seized with the need to repeat the experiment. But I understood that for fun, or out of curiosity in a neuropathic personality or an unstable character, one could succumb to the temptation to repeat the adventure into the unreal.

The legal end of the LSD adventure

Faced with such risks, who could share responsibility for the use made of LSD? The scientists and their experiments, or curious people on all sides (including scientists) who wanted to taste the poisons to egotistically satisfy their misguided consciences?

Sanctions were imposed in two stages, which quickly followed one another. First, Sandoz announced that they would not supply LSD to anybody, not even to doctors or scientists, nor for laboratory research. They had only done so previously with the object of promoting studies, had never marketed the product, and had never made a charge for a single microgram of the substance.

This decision was motivated by press campaigns that for several months had reflected the agitation of social groups from the whole world in the face of the increasing uncontrolled use of LSD, accidents, and tragedies overcoming people who either regularly or occasionally took LSD without medical supervision. Further, the sources of supply of LSD had multiplied; illicit laboratories were now manufacturing the drug for resale traffickers. From the initial interest provoked by an amazing scientific discovery, full of promise, there only remained a dangerous game for minds that were not always sufficiently structured to remain in control of the situation.

The drug finally went underground following its inclusion in List B of narcotics, along with all the other hallucinogens. Scientific investigation was consequently abolished. The law that punishes abuse paralyses research at the same stroke; scientists lose interest in a product associated with drug traffickers and addicts, and that feeds the press with scandals, murders and suicides. The strict prohibition and the end of supply by Sandoz led to suppression of nearly all official experiments controlled by doctors and scientists in hospital research centres.

Psychochemical warfare

At present there are two stocks of LSD in the world. One has a variable, more or less rapid turnover depending on demand, manufactured illegally for those who seek lurid sensations, or believe they are escaping from the society against which they are rebelling. The other stock is fixed, calculated according to strategic requirements, by military forces of different countries who have psychochemical warfare in mind.

The substances called 'incapacitants', of which the leading one is LSD, do not kill, or destroy installations, factories, or lines of communication; but they can paralyse a whole population for hours or a full day, allowing an aggressor to gain occupation without risk, in land that has not been devastated.

The military immediately realized the advantages of such a weapon. The manufacture of LSD is easy and cheap. In a cigarette case a spy or saboteur could carry enough to intoxicate the population of Paris or New York. A large suitcase could hold enough for the whole population of the USA. It would suffice to pulverize the desired quantities with aerosol sprays, or to dissolve them in urban water reservoirs. Identified strategic points would also be contaminated by spies or special agents. Even if the intoxication were not homogeneous, the spectacle of mentally confused people giving themselves over to disorganized and delirious actions would be sufficiently frightening to demoralize those unaffected by the drug.

The picture can be imagined of terrified people in the towns, staggering about, prey to tragic or comic delirium; one can also foresee what such attitudes could trigger off in the streets, industrial and commercial centres, and workplaces. Such commotions would unavoidably lead to accidents, suicides, murders, and all the other catastrophes caused by the human machine running out of control. Ironically, the least distressed would perhaps be those already excluded, isolated and hospitalized for their psychoses. Mentally ill patients are in fact resistant to LSD, and in any case the symptoms resemble those they already have. In the end, the gates of the asylums that protect society from them would then be their protection against those whom the drug has turned mad.

If the reasons guiding the military or states in their preferences for one form of destruction over another can only be understood with difficulty, there is even more scepticism over the humanity of the choice. Compared with the shell, the flamethrower and the atom bomb, what should one think of bacteriological warfare and mind poisons like LSD? The issue of disarmament, even if it were resolved, would only serve as a mask for the more difficult to control biological and chemical weapons.

A balance sheet

If one had to draw up a balance sheet for the discovery of LSD, the fact that its use might be restricted to the military or to those who are unhappy is regrettable. For LSD remains, in spite of everything, a remarkable research tool for analysing and understanding the human mind during normal and pathological activity. Through its capacity to reproduce all varieties of mental illness in their acute forms, and all kinds of visionary states, LSD could have rendered immense services. Not only, with this substance, can one carry out objective studies on mental anomalies set off voluntarily; but the psychiatrist, the psychologist, and all those working in mental illness and with patients suffering from it, can experience with LSD, from the inside, the delirium and hallucinations that they only see in mentally ill patients from the outside.

If one also follows certain philosophers, analysts or poets, hallucinogens such as LSD can help in understanding the mechanisms of artistic and even scientific creation, by analysing the mechanism of associations and their artistic, literary or scientific expression.

Who could deny that better understanding of the mind's infrastructure is useful? We can never know well enough what we are, and LSD remains a key; a pass that can open the door behind which all our inhibitions lie locked away. This is why LSD does not set free or provide anything other than what is already present in the human mind, but in allowing the extraction and presentation of what is in the brain in a new way, it should teach us many other things. For the first time, we can empty ourselves of our mind, project it into a transitory state of 'out of mind' to have it dissected alive by others, and at the end, when the experiment is finished, replace and reconstruct our consciousness with a brain now capable of sorting out our sensations and inhibiting all useless perceptions. As long as LSD and the hallucinogens are blacklisted by law, and because of the use that traffickers and drug addicts make of them, such explorations and studies remain impossible.

The interests of society and science reside neither in total prohibition nor in a complete absence of legal protection. But to whom should the studies on LSD and the other hallucinogens be entrusted? To scientists, doctors, philosophers or artists? Who shall say? There are no bad drugs, only good and bad users or prescribers of these drugs.

Our inclinations, in disturbed times, are perhaps not conducive to an equitable use in terms of risk and safety. Equally, who can say that in times of peace such experiments would not give rise to insecurity and distress? Thus we have lost the right to use these possibly dangerous instruments for clarifying the mysteries of mental illness and insanity. We shall see now how without understanding the mechanism of storms of insanity, we have nevertheless begun to try to calm them.

The beginnings of psychochemistry

Fabricating mental illness with elixirs such as LSD helped neither the mental patient nor the doctor, because each had acquired a diabolical partner, whose mysterious treachery they had been unable to master. On the contrary, a harmful current had diverted the interest of their experiments, turning them against one another, for a dangerous contagion had developed amongst the poor souls who thought they could find a new paradise in what was but an infernal antechamber.

Back at square one, the psychiatrists were once more trying out all the possible combinations of their therapeutic games.

I have scruples in talking about 'games' to describe therapeutic research in psychiatry in the 1950s, and some would criticize me for naming attempts to cure mental illness in this way. Does it matter? We wanted to be doctors, in this non-medical science that psychiatry then was. Outside our administrative obligations to admit and restrain the patients, and to take care of their security and physical hygiene, therapeutic psychiatry was only a game—a purely gratuitous activity that in the mind of the player has no objective other than the pleasure it provides. This was the case for many psychiatrists who tried a few treatments, analysed and described the symptoms, and arranged them to construct a methodological classification of mental illness. The desire to cure was a secondary consideration, for, apart from shock therapies with well-defined indications, the result was a fortunate or unfortunate throw of the dice, which settled very little.

Nevertheless, some of us still cherished the hope of finding drugs that would be effective in mental disorders.

The psychotonic amines

The amines, organic compounds derived from ammonia, include products that have a particular affinity for the nervous system, principally the amphetamines—also called waking amines, psychamines or psychotonic amines. Until recent years their prescription was unrestricted; they were included in products intended to combat fatigue and sleep. One of their secondary effects was to combat appetite. Taking these substances gave a feeling of euphoria, enhanced lucidity, increased capacity for work, and improvement of memory, and many schoolchildren and students revising for examinations and competitions used them to increase their intellectual output. In fact, it was a matter of subjective impressions, for true work and performances were not improved, as could be appreciated when controls were carried out on volunteers using psychological tests. However, the actions of these amphetamines was perceived by those who took them as a mental and physical comfort, providing ease and intellectual ability, and also a feeling of enhanced physical stamina.

Not only used for their psychiatric properties, the amphetamines were also thought to increase physical effort capacity, and were given to athletes and to soldiers before battle. I have not been able to verify whether the European armies in the Second World War made use of amphetamines or methylamphetamines (in France these products were called Maxiton and Tonedron), but Japanese friends have told me how they were used in the training camps at Kyushu where 'kamikaze' crews were being set up.

From 1944 the Japanese, under pressure from the American forces who were little by little regaining the Pacific strategic positions, had recruited volunteer soldiers to fight till the death in hopeless battles. Suicide aeroplanes were manufactured, of basic construction allowing only for the transport of bombs and explosives as far as the target, with a reduced supply of fuel to make sure the flight was one way—for the aeroplane and pilot's mission was solely to crash on the intended target, whether a factory, troops or a warship.

The pilots of these aeroplanes, all volunteers, were trained in camps where an atmosphere was created intended to maintain the combative momentum for these suicide missions. In recognition of the exaltation of their patriotic faith, and the agreed sacrifice of dying for their country, a game licence was provided: freedom for all passions. Restrictions were abolished for these heroes, who were given abundant food, paid courtesans, unlimited alcohol, and, in order to maintain their psychic excitement, regularly increasing doses of amphetamines—in particular, methylamphetamines (methamphetamines).

Administered orally or intravenously, amphetamine gives a feeling of well-being, excitement, and physical and mental strength, without hallucination or loss of self-control. When the doses are taken by groups of people, a reciprocal excitement spreads from one individual to another, sustaining a general climate of euphoria, desire for pleasure, or for immediate action. If it is true that the overall outcome is not greatly influenced, the hyperactivity provoked by the drug is obvious, as can be seen in the course of rock concerts where the band and spectators are united in an enthusiasm that sometimes degenerates into a destructive fury.

The use of amphetamines expanded in Japan after the war, so much so that this country was the first to introduce prohibitive legislation concerning these products.

I confess to having been surprised to hear of these misplaced uses of waking amines, for in Europe we were only acquainted with their use as stimulants, or in association with aspirin to combat influenza, or coryza, unblock the nose, or prevent sleep. It is precisely this virtue of counteracting sleep that doctors exploit to reawaken patients who have accidentally or deliberately taken barbiturates, hypnotics, or sedatives in toxic doses, from their coma.

From narcoanalysis to amphetamine shock

When an individual is drugged, voluntarily or not, with phenobarbitone or any other powerful hypnotic, sleep ensues, and this sleep, increasingly profound, ends in a coma, which must be ended at all costs. Stomach wash-out, if performed in time, is sometimes enough, and little by little consciousness returns. This phase of returning to the waking state is often accompanied by speech, at first incoherent, then clearer, and sometimes these patients go on to talk uninhibitedly about events, explain their behaviour, and try to understand their actions. What was said spontaneously did not escape the doctors who were overseeing their patient's reawakening, and they found material of use in effective psychotherapy in these monologues. Indeed, during the return to consciousness, the patient, half-asleep, felt free from the barriers and obstacles formed by conscious or unconscious emotional constraints in the family or social environment. The return from the depths of the coma coincided with memories and reminiscences that freed the patient, enabling long-buried memories to be recalled and got rid of with relief.

Each of us has experienced some of these involuntary sentences that have escaped during sleep from a relative, friend or spouse, whose secret is overheard, sometimes inquisitively. The involuntary talking of the dreamer and sleeper does not always result in an indiscretion or a catastrophic confession, but sometimes it results in liberation from an oppressive psychological burden.

One would like to consider these things said in semi-consciousness and let out spontaneously as 'moments of truth'. Hence the name 'truth drug' improperly given to thiopentone sodium (Pentothal), the intravenous injection of which, in average doses, leads to a semi-sleep during which the patient is questioned.

The psychiatrist exploited this stage of psychological vagueness with verbiage in the course of reawakening from coma, by provoking it artificially under the name of 'narcoanalysis'. Unlike Freudian psychoanalysis, which is carried out in wide-awake individuals, narcoanalysis is performed with the patient in a state of incomplete sleep (subnarcosis) following an intravenous injection of thiopentone sodium or amylobarbitone (Amytal). The psychotherapeutic investigation of the subconscious can then use information supplied by the patient while half-asleep. From experience I can state that the expression 'truth drug' applied to Pentothal is entirely inappropriate, for malingerers, liars and story-tellers are quite capable of telling falsehoods or making up stories during subnarcosis; it depends on the degree of permeation of the brain by the product, as well as on the psychological make-up of the individual. At any rate, a judicial test to obtain a confession has nothing to do with the medical standpoint, where the only object is to relieve patients of their problems, even at the expense of lies or fantasizing that are externalized and which are a useful way of analysing the patient's personality.

Overdoses and suicide attempts with barbiturates had thus led to the introduction of a psychiatric therapeutic procedure—narcoanalysis. These same comas were also to lead to the discovery of another method of exploring the psyche, using amphetamines as 'waking amines'. In cases of barbiturate overdoses, gastric wash-out was not effective when the poison had already entered the blood and permeated the brain and nerve centres: an antidote was therefore needed. Amphetamine was found to be a very effective counter-poison, which could be given intravenously in up to ten, twenty, or even fifty times the dose usually given to wake patients from a coma.

Those who first experimented with this method realized that at the time of its action, when the amphetamine roused the sleeper, the reawakening was accompanied by a euphoria, which contrasted with the depression provoking the suicidal impulse. After the injection, the patient would become loquacious, voluntarily recounting facts and anecdotes, and displaying an excitement, which was sometimes aggressive. This attitude, associated with easy and cheerful speech, sometimes gave way to sudden anguish with freeing of suppressed emotion, which seemed to relieve the patient. With stronger doses, given to consolidate the reawakening, there could be an outburst of acute mania.

This is how the psychiatrists came to think of using amphetamines, to provoke in patients what was called 'amphetamine shock', characterized by the phenomena described above. This 'amphetamine shock' was achieved by the intravenous injection of methylamphetamine, a synthetic compound more active than amphetamine. After the injection, immediately followed by cardiac acceleration and a burst of psychological excitement, some tensed-up, reticent patients, inhibited in their behaviour and thought processes, showed a desire to speak, and to talk about themselves, facilitating analysis and counselling by the psychotherapist.

It is perhaps this 'high', analogous in its release to that provoked by heroin but very different in its manifestations, which has seduced the 'speed freaks'—amphetamine addicts who derived from it excitement, an inflated personality, and a sought-after passion to live beyond the prohibitions and barriers of society. Artificial courage, expansive goodwill, explosive energy, contempt for the law, are what amphetamines provide for modern-day kamikazes.

Here again, the gap widens between the doctor's therapeutic aims and the use the amateur makes of the drug, first unwittingly, soon all too well-informed, and later established in a permanent drug addiction.

I will not linger to describe amphetamine addicts, any more than to analyse the other manifestations of the use and abuse of the various psychological drugs leading to addiction, as I wish to confine myself to describing my experience with medicines for the mind. However, I cannot resist the desire to give an account of the adventure of this doctor, to whom, of course, I give an imaginary name.

A car that gets high

In the fishing tackle department at the Samaritaine, Max Cory had asked for some sea fishing reels. As the shop assistant asked him to clarify to her what kind of fish he wanted to catch, he first said he did not know, then, bursting with laughter, 'Sperm whales, sharks, whales, big fish, whatever!'

The employee, who did not greatly appreciate the reply, showed him the biggest she had, and Max Cory said, 'I'll take three.'

He then bought rods, hundreds of metres of nylon, eel nets, fitted hooks, lures of all kinds, and lead weights of all sizes.

'Are you going far to fish?' asked the employee at the packing desk, who had parcelled up the twenty-three purchases.

'In the Creuse, near Éguzon,' answered Cory.

'Why did you buy all your equipment for sea fishing?' innocently asked the salesgirl, who was waiting at the check-out with the list of purchases to be paid for. Cory, who was writing a cheque, raised his eyes towards his questioner and with all the seriousness in the world replied:

'Last year, while we were having a picnic, I inadvertently threw the salt-cellar into the dam.'

This time the salesgirl consented to laugh, and called a store assistant to help Max Cory carry his purchases to his car.

'This won't go inside,' said the employee in front of the 4CV already crammed with packets, boxes and brightly coloured blankets.

'Oh, yes it will,' said Cory. He flattened the boxes by stamping on them, broke the rods, crushed the packets, forced the doors, and took the wheel after having given the employee an enormous tip.

'Cheers, friend!'

The 4CV started up with difficulty, but finally moved away, backfiring. Cory took the Pont-Neuf direction, without bothering about the traffic lights.

A policeman blew his whistle, tried to pick out the car's registration num-ber, gave this up; the 4CV was already as far up as the Vert-Galant statue.

'Stupid, this "no entry" along the rue Dauphine!' grumbled Cory.

The rue Guénégaud was already blocked.

'Too bad, this will be shorter.'

The 4CV was facing a red 'no entry' traffic sign, but the rue Dauphine was clear and Cory entered it. He passed astonished drivers who made signals to him, and soon found himself in front of a bus.

'Go back!' cried Cory, 'I'm in a hurry. I'm going to the hospital!'

The bus driver of course did not move, and hooted his horn. Cory got out of his 4CV, and, indifferent to the crowd that was beginning to collect, repeated his command to the bus driver.

'Go back. I am going to the hospital!'

Faced with the immobility of the huge vehicle, the gibes of the crowd and the threats of the bus driver, Cory got back behind the wheel of his 4CV, started it up, and began to reverse. The bus driver also started up, the crowd of gaping onlookers began to disperse, everyone thinking that the 4CV and its driver had given up the struggle. Not a bit of it. Cory had gone back to take a run, and drove straight at the bus.

'There we go, my beautiful, he's the one who's going to be smashed in!'

The 4CV crashed into the bumper of the bus. Cory was thrown out onto the road through the door which had burst open. His head struck the kerbstone at the edge of the gutter and he lost consciousness . . .

A police rescue van took the wounded man from the rue Dauphine to the Hôtel-Dieu. An X-ray confirmed that he did not have a fracture, but he was kept in for observation. During the night, Max Cory got up, and the nurses saw him in his nightshirt at the bedside of the patients, taking their pulses, checking their temperature charts, giving them drinks, and call-ing for medicines for them. He was so unruly that the duty house doctor was called, and he sent him to the manic ward. In every hospital, in those days, this was the dumping ground for drunken tramps and other brawl-ing and exuberant manic people. In this special department, either they calmed down and went out, or they did not improve and were sent to Sainte-Anne.

Provided with the appropriate certificate, I admitted Max Cory three days after his accident.

'My dear colleague, I am the victim of an arbitrary compulsory admis-sion. I must go urgently to the American Hospital where my mother-in-law is having an operation this morning. Let me get out right away—my wife is waiting for me.'

'My dear colleague, you must calm down a bit. You have had a road traffic accident, but it seems you were not in a normal state. Your mother-in-law is in my office, and it is your wife who has just had a miscarriage at the American Hospital. I immediately reassure you she is getting on very well. But as for you, tell me a little about your history.'

'I will tell you everything you want, but give me ten or so Maxiton tablets, or put me to sleep.'

I did indeed, put Dr Cory to sleep, and two weeks later, we shook hands when he left the hospital. In the meantime, he had given me his story.

Newly set up in a surgery he had started in the western suburbs of Paris, the young and likeable Dr Cory quickly built up a large practice. Day and night, devoted and tireless, he coped well with overworking, helped by his young wife and a Spanish maid. Then, during the winter, he developed a heavy dose of 'flu, followed by sinusitis, not bad enough to keep him at home, but resistant to antibiotics. After the acute phase, persistent migraine attacks started up. So here is our Dr Max full up with aspirin, then Corydrane, to overcome his fatigue. No question of stopping with a new practice. He had to keep going. Corydrane is aspirin with an ephedrine derivative—a stimulant. At night, when he had an urgent call, he had a Maxiton or Tonedron (amphetamines) to keep him awake. This prevented fatigue and sleep. Requests for appointments were not declined, and built up; ten, twenty, thirty, and more. Sylviane Cory and young Pilar are themselves also upset by the work, especially by Max's agitation, increasingly excited, increasingly snowed under with work, but whose pace and zest stimulate, encourage and comfort the patients.

'Sylviane, you are tired. Look, take a tablet. You see. It will buck you up. We must keep going, blow it!'

The samples of Maxiton, Tonedron and Corydrane which Max requests from the drug companies are not enough. At this time these drugs can be bought freely, without a prescription. The dose taken had to be increased at all costs, and Max's outlook extended to his wife and the maid. Pilar is also taking Maxiton, and Dr Cory's villa is now a festive palace; a place of shadowy characters where everyone is restless, excited, and more and more agitated. A few patients seem to be surprised by the excessive zeal of their good Dr Cory, but he makes accurate diagnoses, has a sure hand, and is kind, if talkative; he explains everything that is wrong. He takes great care. Then, one night:

'Do you know, Max, I think I am pregnant.'

For Sylviane this is wonderful; for him, it is a catastrophe, a stroke of bad luck.

'It's too early, too quick. We'll manage, you've made a mistake. Here, take this.'

The round of tablets goes on. Sylviane and little Pilar are anxiously and impatiently awaiting the holiday they are going to have in the Creuse near Éguzon. But Max falls by the wayside; he is now swallowing tablets in tens and getting others to do so too—his wife—the maid—and also the patients.

'It'll be fine, fine. We must hold on. We'll go fishing in the Éguzon dam, I will take you back under the chestnut trees in the Noire valley where you used to read *La Petite Fadette* to me. Here, take your dose of tablets;

here is Pilar's. I won't be in for lunch, I'll go to the Samar to buy some fishing tackle.'

The 4CV runs badly: it ought to be traded in. It too is exhausted, worn out; it has had its day. It also needs some stimulant, and before it 'freaks out' Max Cory, in his delirium, is going to dope it, the 'poor old lady'.

'When you think, sir, that not only did I swallow fifty Maxiton tablets a day, that I got my wife and the maid to take at least ten, but that each morning I poured a box into the tank of my katchevo!'

Max Cory is pale and thin, but all that is but a bad memory. The 'katchevo' gave up the ghost against the bus, Sylviane is at Éguzon at her mother's home, and Pilar is having her two months holiday at Pamplona with her family.

'She wanted us to go there for the San Fermin, because of the bull-fights, the finest in Spain. But this year it will be Éguzon again. Next year perhaps?'

Max Cory, with a smile on his lips, looked at me, 'The bulls, the bull-fight . . . if you gave amphetamines to the bulls, and the toreadors!'

Incorrigible Dr Cory . . .

So, around the 1950s, between narcoanalysis with amylobarbitone and shock with methylamphetamine, patients walked between two syringes along the road of 'biological therapeutics', where shock and psychosurgical measures now competed with a completely new psycho-chemistry. The hallucinogens (mescaline, LSD) used in experimental deliriums, the barbiturates in the semi-comatose sleep of narcoanalysis and methylamphetamine in the psychological outburst of amphetamine shock constituted a pharmacopoeia of active drugs for us, of which we tried to make good use. We also used some soft drugs; so soft that they hardly did anything, but which had very pretty names.

From intelligence amino acid to succinic dinitrile

In spite of his taste for philosophy and his knowledge of psychology, Jean Delay remained very much a doctor. Unlike his colleagues in the asylums, he was cast in the mould of the Health and Social Security ser-vices, rooted in medical science and therapeutics. It is no coincidence, therefore, that great discoveries in modern psychiatric therapeutics and in psychopharmacology should have been made in his department at Sainte-Anne, or very quickly assessed, developed and improved. Attracted by everything that could help or cure, he had very quickly used shock therapies, of which, with Soulairac, he described the biological syndrome. Prudently, he had had lobotomies performed by Puech, but with no less reserve and diplomacy he withdrew from this psychosurgical route. On the other hand, chemical therapeutics—psychochemistry—greatly interested him, and when he was asked to try glutamic acid in mentally retarded patients, he did so without hesitation. This is how, with

Pierre Pichot, he was able to show that this amino acid promoted psychological performance (measured by means of mental tests) in some oligophrenic patients (learning-challenged). And as Jean Delay prided himself, and rightly so, on writing well (he liked to coin clear expressions and precise neologisms), he named glutamic acid the 'intelligence amino acid'. The term made a fortune, as did the drug company that then sold the product under the name of 'Glutaminol'. All French youngsters took it before examinations.

Delay believed in chemical therapeutics, and when he was also asked to study the dinitriles on some patients, he willingly agreed. The use of dinitriles arose from the work of two Swedes, Hyden and Artelius, who had found that malonic dinitrile stimulated production of ribonucleotides in the cerebral nerve cells. They had successfully tested this product, they said, in mentally ill patients.

The nitriles are more or less toxic (hydrocyanic acid, a deadly poison, is a nitrile) and malonic dinitrile is sufficiently so for its administration to bring on the beginnings of a coma, from which the patient was lifted by giving an antidote with a sodium hyposulphite base.

Delay had given two of his pupils, Deniker and Sizaret, the task of applying Hyden and Artelius's treatment. They confined themselves to a few experiments, for the procedure was not very practicable because of increased risk and variable results. They were getting ready to abandon the treatment, which was in a way merely a chemical coma treatment, when Dr Debat's laboratory, which had prepared the product they were giving, suggested replacing the malonic dinitrile with the less dangerous succinic dinitrile, which was put up in ampoules and called Suxil. The effectiveness of a medication is often—but not always—directly proportional to its toxicity, and in this case there was as much difference between malonic dinitrile and succinic dinitrile as between the poison hydrocyanic acid and cherry-laurel water, which contains traces of it and is prescribed for coughs. In spite of this, Suxil for a while appeared helpful in mild depression. In those days, double-blind controlled trials were not done.

Even if Suxil added nothing more to Delay's reputation, it was not completely without interest. For if I now recall the Suxil adventure, which nearly everybody has now forgotten, the concept of stimulating ribonucleic acid (RNA) remains today the hypothesis for the most stimulating research in the study of brain medication. RNA is a key constituent in the genetic mechanism; and the same Swede Holgar Hyden at the University of Gothenburg had, in the 1970s, front-page coverage in the press by declaring that it might be possible one day to control thought by producing molecular changes in active brain substances. Now modified RNA could in its turn alter the fundamental substance of cerebral cells, and consequently their functioning and thus the mental state. Holgar Hyden now no longer speaks of malonic dinitrile, but of tricyanoaminopropene.

This substance would have had the effect of making people more suggestible. Straightaway, politicians, essayists and novelists drew hasty conclusions and enjoyed imagining the uses which state police could make of substances like tricyanoaminopropene, which would only have to be put in the drinking water for a whole population to be conditioned through induced chemical suggestibility. Tricyanoaminopropene is still a nitrile, and Holgar Hyden shows great perseverance in his scientific convictions.

As for me, I do not think that the brain's 'magicians' dawn' is yet near, but a day will perhaps come when luck will favour not the necessity but a desire that I decline to judge because in this particular case it does not seem necessary to me for human happiness.

At any rate, these nitriles, to which I wish neither good nor evil, I do consider very active on the evidence of my personal experiments, recalling that iminodipropionitrile (IDPN), which enabled me to develop the turning mice which I have mentioned earlier, itself also belonged to the same chemical family.

Curare relaxation

The term 'relaxation' oddly enough has a somatic predominance in French and a psychological predominance in English. Usage has resulted in one more anglicism being added to our language, and so if we consult the dictionaries a hotchpotch is suggested, which common use has adopted. 'To relax oneself' *Robert's Dictionary* tells us, means to calm down, to rest physically and intellectually. In this way one can draw a parallel between the suppression or diminution in contraction of a muscle and the dissipation or reduction in the psychological tension of an anguished or anxious person. When, today, you say to somebody 'Relax!', everyone understands. To illustrate this passage from contracted muscle to calmed mind, I will continue with a story about experimental medicine.

Why did I agree to choose a patient for Monsieur Lapique and Julian de Ajuriaguerra that afternoon in the autumn of 1946? Why? It was Ajuria who asked me to.

'We need a volunteer patient, young, who would not be very suggestible. It is for a curarization. Monsieur Lapique wants to see a curarization.'

Who was Monsieur Lapique? Who is de Ajuriaguerra? What is a curarization?

If you look in an encyclopaedia you will see that Lapique was a French physiologist who was born at Épinal in 1866 and died in Paris in 1952. You will also read that he defined and measured nerve excitability by a constant which he called a *chronaxie*. There is no point in knowing what a chronaxie is, as it no longer serves much purpose, but for my tale it is good to know that Lapique was a member of the Academy of Medicine from 1925 and of the Academy of Science from 1930. Lapique was eighty years old in 1946: he was what is called a great scientist, and he wanted to see a curarization in man.

In your encyclopaedia you will not find the name of Dr Julian de Ajuriaguerra, although he was then a professor at the College of France. Of Spanish origin, this young neurologist and psychiatrist had been welcomed at Sainte-Anne, where in 1946, in parallel with Henri Ey, he instructed us in discriminating and outstanding neurology in the purest tradition of Jules Dejerine and Joseph Babinsky. Ajuria, as we called him familiarly, was more a friend and comrade than a master, and none of the house doctors at Sainte-Anne could ever refuse him anything.

Finally, if you open your encyclopaedia again (but perhaps you would not need to) you will find under the word 'curare' that it is a poison of blackish colour, extracted from various plants that the tribes of tropical South America use to poison their arrows. You might also read the following quotation from our great Claude Bernard: 'Curare causes death by destruction of all the motor neurones, without affecting the sensory nerves'—which is only partially correct.

So, between the two scientists who wanted to inject a paralysing poison into a mental patient, what was I to do in this awkward situation?

Most surprisingly, I knew nothing about it myself. In short, I wanted to please Ajuria, who wanted to please Monsieur Lapique, who wanted to give himself the pleasure of curarizing a human being, whereas his illustrious predecessor Claude Bernard had only curarized frogs, rabbits and dogs.

Here again, I raise the difficult problem of medical experimentation, its justification before the law, ethics and therapeutic progress. Admittedly, it was not the arrow poison that was going to be injected, but a purified extract of the active alkaloid, well-defined chemically: d-tubocurarine. The exact dose needed for a non-fatal curarization was known. In the event of prolonged respiratory paralysis, it would be enough to perform artificial respiration, with oxygen inhalation, while waiting calmly for everything to turn out right. Nevertheless, to validate this trial in a pragmatic way, in my mind there needed to be a serious motive such as research or possible therapeutic application. This is what I was waiting to learn with curiosity and interest.

As Ajuria had told me that he only hoped to obtain muscular relaxation, I had thought of using a patient who presented a severe form of stuporous melancholy, so that all his motor activity was inhibited. Absorbed in sadness, he no longer paid any interest to his surroundings; he seemed not to hear, and apart from a few groans, he remained dumb, withdrawn, with his arms pressed against his chest, and his neck stiff.

It was not easy to get this patient to lie on the examination couch, and hold his arm for the curare injection, which Ajuria gave very slowly into a vein.

He had worked out a mild dose, but the patient had lost weight through frequently refusing food, and the curarization developed very quickly. It first affected his neck, which he held flexed onto his chest, until his head slowly tilted backwards to rest on the pillow. A strange astonishment came into his eyes, a fleeting look of inexpressible surprise, but quickly his eyelids dropped, which is the first sign of curarization. After a few flickerings of the eyelashes the eyes finally closed at the same time as the jaws unclenched, leaving the mouth half-open; then the arms and legs, which two nurses were holding, relaxed. Soon, lying on the white sheet, instead of a contracted, taut, almost convulsed individual, we had a flaccid, flabby body not only incapable of moving a hand, arm or foot, but unable even to raise his eyelids. The patient's respiration had slowed and diminished in amplitude. Keeping an eye on this, as well as on the pulse, ready to intervene with an oxygen respirator, I watched my two neurologists, who, indifferent to the secondary psychological effects of this curarization, merely analysed the neurological signs with an attitude that did shock me a little.

I am not going to make excuses for them, for I have always felt indignant when doctors, out of confessed or unconscious egotism, forget the person within the patient, with no feeling for the drama of their illness, merely to satisfy their impassioned curiosity.

Lapique descended onto the limp puppet which my patient had become, and passively moved his arms and legs, which he lifted up then let fall back on the bed. Ajuria had handed him a reflex hammer with which he struck the Achilles and patellar tendons to see if the reflexes were still present. Bending over the inert subject, the elderly scientist palpated the atonic, limp muscle masses with his gnarled hands. This limp body interested him as if he had been palpating the anatomy of a puppet, and when he had thoroughly massaged him he straightened up.

'Perfect. The whole body is paralysed. Let us now see about sensation.'

He had taken from the lapel of his jacket, behind his rosette of the Legion of Honour, a long pin inserted into the lining, and again approaching the body, he pricked the legs, thighs, and abdomen, all the while watching the patient's inert face. In spite of the pain, the latter could not react by wincing because all his muscles were paralysed. Lapique increased his pressure on the pin, which he forced a good millimetre into the skin of one thigh. The patient, who was barely breathing, took a deeper breath, and a long groan came from his half-open lips. A smile lit up the face of the old doctor.

'Obviously! He feels everything,' he declared, and once more scraping the soles of the patient's feet without eliciting any reflex, he replaced his faithful needle behind his rosette.

As he was putting his overcoat back on, preparing to leave, I asked him:

'What's going to happen to the patient? How long will his paralysis last? What should I do?'

Ajuria reassured me, 'There's nothing to do. He'll come round in a few minutes.'

It was 'to see' that Lapique had come. He wanted to 'see' a curariza-tion.

'Thank you my old friend. Goodbye.'

Lapique did not even thank me. Muttering a few words to Ajuriaguerra he went out rubbing his hands with satisfaction—unless it was to warm his numb limbs; it was a cold day.

I stayed with the two male nurses near my patient's still inert body, anxious to see him take a normal breath and regain the use of his limbs. As his eyelids were flickering a little, I lifted them, to observe that his look was not too anguished, but showed great astonishment. As his respira-tions were still short, I got him to inhale a little oxygen. I did not know at the time that a curare antidote derived from the calabar bean could have decurarized my patient within a few minutes. I still wonder if Ajuria and Lapique knew about the antagonists eserine (physostigmine) and neostigmine. At any rate, they didn't mention them to me.

Little by little the patient began to move; he now kept his eyes open and shifted his arms and legs. When he managed to sit on the edge of the bed, he only maintained this position for a few seconds, then col-lapsed back.

'I am very tired,' he murmured.

A nurse drew my attention to the fact that this was the first sentence spoken by the patient for many weeks. Normally dumb, he only responded to questions with groans.

'What have you done to me? I feel heavy, as if my body weighed tons.'

Our dumb patient was speaking. His anxiety remained, but the grave stuporous stage of his condition and his contracted bearing had given way, following the atonia provoked by the curare. This unexpected and beneficial result gave me the additional satisfaction of having carried out a therapeutic procedure that had escaped the two neurologists, who had only been concerned with the single paralysing action of curare. Further-more, I felt exonerated from guilt about the wanton act they had made me commit: I had discovered that a useful psychological relaxation could be achieved by curarization.

From infracurarization to the first tranquillizers

Coincidences and luck have often managed to find me: perhaps because I knew how to make use of them. However, it must not be thought that everything happens at the first throw of the dice.

Encouraged by the improved behaviour of the patient after one curarization, I gave him some more, lighter ones, which did not improve his condition any further. The melancholy he presented was of a severe form, resistant even to electroconvulsion. Moreover, curarization was not easy to put into general use, and carried some risks. Curare began to be used solely to facilitate the work of the surgeon, who could operate better when muscles were relaxed. Only competent anaesthetists such as Pierre Huguenard, and pioneer surgeons, performed curarizations, surrounded by watchful staff and sophisticated apparatus. So I gave up curarizing depressed patients, feeling that psychological calming and relaxation did not warrant running the risk of generalized muscle paralysis from curare. It was then that another set of coincidences happened, which I will enumerate in order:

1   First, chemists had tried to make synthetic curare because obtaining and purifying natural curares was not easy.
2   To be active, these synthetic curares had to have a chemical formula containing two quadruply substituted nitrogen atoms known as 'quaternary ammonium compounds'.
3   All quaternary ammonium compounds were not curarizants, but they all paralysed the sympathetic ganglia, and for this reason were called 'ganglioplegics'.
4   Finally, doctors had noticed that these ganglioplegics, which were destroyed by the gastric digestive juices, were active by the rectal route, as suppositories.

Of course, psychiatric doctors trying all new treatments had tried ganglioplegic suppositories in certain mental illnesses, but without success.

If you have followed steps 1 to 4, we will go back to it in reverse to explain to you *why I gave curare by the rectal route*. My reasoning was as follows:

If ganglioplegics administered to mental patients were ineffective, perhaps this was because they were not strong enough. Amongst the ganglioplegics, the strongest have a curarizing activity. The synthetic curares are very ganglioplegic, but the natural ones are even more so. So, let us try out the ganglioplegic properties of the natural curares.

It is possible to dissociate ganglioplegic from curarizing activity, since it was known that the curares are not active by the oral route. Indeed, the Indians eat the game they have killed with their curare-coated arrows quite safely. So I could, by administering curares by the rectum (at the end of the digestive tract) eliminate any risk of curarization, retaining the ganglioplegic strength of the natural curares.

For good measure, I had suppositories made up of *d*-tubocurarine in a large dose.

The first person to whom I administered a curare suppository was an alcoholic patient who had been weaned off alcohol for several weeks but who had developed depression at the thought of going back to work. He had not got over the distress and anxiety that came over him when thinking about returning to his family and to his comrades who knew the circumstances of his compulsory admission in a bout of delirium tremens. Worried and agitated, he was always fidgeting, and nothing could pacify him or restore his morale.

I had explained to the nurses who gave out the medicines that there were some new suppositories, and asked them to let me know whether they were well tolerated.

I was starting to write up the patients' notes when a nurse came looking for me.

'Something strange has happened to Monsieur Lep: he has just gone to bed and says he cannot move.'

I rushed to the room where I found the patient stretched out, his eyes closed, but calm and relaxed. He explained to me that five minutes after inserting his suppository, he suddenly felt very heavy and was overcome by acute fatigue. He turned round towards his bed, and laid down.

'My eyes are closed, but I am not asleep. It is curious; I feel heavier and heavier.'

This was the first phase of curarization, which has a superficial effect and relaxes the muscles a little, and which is known as the atonic phase of Bremer (who described it). Contrary to what I—and everyone else—thought, the curare could be absorbed through the lower digestive tract. The curare was active by the rectal route.

Suddenly I felt frightened, because I remembered that the dose of curare in the suppository represented at least ten times the active intravenous dose. I immediately asked for the oxygen cylinder and mask, and had a neostigmine injection prepared. I was quickly reassured, however, for the curarization by the rectal route was only an infracurarization. To paralyse, curare (natural or synthetic) must permeate the points at which it acts at a certain concentration that depends upon the rate of absorption and diffusion of the product. Now the absorption of curare is rapid by the intravenous route, and nil by the gastric route, because it is destroyed in the stomach and intestine, and slow by the rectal route, where absorption is very gradual.

And so this patient remained stretched out for more than an hour on his bed, without his muscular relaxation at any time becoming a true curare paralysis. At the same time, he experienced an undoubted psychological calming, contemporaneous with his atony, and after completely recovering all his muscular strength, he dropped off to sleep.

When I reported my observations first to Jean Delay, then to René Hazard and Jean Cheymol, the same reservations greeted my remarks. Since Claude Bernard, it was common knowledge that the curares were not active rectally. To make what I had found credible, I had to demonstrate it *a posteriori* in an animal, using a nerve–muscle preparation, with curarizations produced in rabbits with tiny curare suppositories. I had papers published in France and abroad explaining this technique, and the American journal *Science* agreed to publish a note with illustrations of the experiment.

This method of psychological relaxation with curare suppositories had appeared at first to be a little risky to doctors who were overawed by this formidable poison, but after recognizing its harmlessness, many used it successfully in mild depression associated with anxiety. Patent preparations were marketed with natural curare and synthetic curare too. One of these was manufactured under the name of Isocurine.

Curarization by the rectal route, which in fact was merely infracurarization, an enforced muscle relaxation, interested many scientific and medical circles. I received copious correspondence on the subject of this psychosomatic application of curare. Already the problem of synthetic relaxants was giving rise to much research. I was not the only one to have discovered that muscular relaxation produced by a medication is accompanied by a psychological relaxation. The year I discovered infracurarization by the rectal route, mephenesin, a muscular relaxant acting via the medullary pathway, was marketed under the name of Décontractyl.

Décontractyl, first used by athletes for muscles stiffened through exertion, was also used for anxious and depressed patients; it was a chemical derivative of propanediol, from which one day the first tranquillizer was to come, destined to extend throughout the world: meprobamate, also called Equanil and Miltown.

During the 1950s all psychological research tackled from the point of view of relaxation, either with curare or with medullary paralysing agents, was abandoned for a time in favour of a cardinal discovery, whose importance the general public has still not appreciated. This discovery, as important as that of antibiotics, represented a more significant advance than that of cardiac surgery, renal transplantation and other organ grafts. It liberated millions of patients incarcerated in psychiatric asylums. Medically speaking, it made a mental life possible again for healthy bodies paralysed by a sick brain.

Chlorpromazine, a neuroleptic medication, in 1952 became the first chemical treatment for the psychoses. From this fundamental discovery were to follow many others, which in the course of ten years of psychopharmacological research transformed not only the treatment, but also the public image, of mental illness.

3
Discovery of the neuroleptics

Manoeuvres

To understand a story

Collision between two bodies, inanimate or living, means the loss of sustained momentum, or the freezing of a vital force. From this clash springs a struggle lost by one and won by the other. Between the success and failure of the encounter exists 'shock', which can take many forms. States of shock, physical or psychological, provide many surprises.

For lack of therapeutic measures, the psychiatrist used shocks to set free captive minds trapped within the mental illness, but for other doctors shock is something to be feared.

'The operation was a success, but the patient did not stand up to the operative/anaesthetic shock . . .' this sentence, spoken by the surgeon or the resuscitation anaesthetist—how many times have we heard it? This contradiction between the state of shock dreaded by the surgeon, and the psychological shock paradoxically wished for and even provoked by the psychiatrist, was to be resolved by one of the greatest therapeutic advances of the middle of the century.

The story of this invention, arising in France, is not simple; foreign exegetes have often only analysed the memories of biased protagonists or unedited technical leaflets from pharmaceutical laboratories. Having lived through this adventure, I can relate the story with the authority of my long experience of the development of psychiatric therapeutics and the fact that I was working with the principal players in the discovery, all of whom I know and who were all still very much alive at the time of writing.

More curares

The curares, which had interested me on account of the psychological relaxation they provided, were even more interesting to surgeons and anaesthetists. Indeed, relaxed muscles are essential to successful surgery; access to the operative field is easier, and when the wound has to be closed and sutured it is easier to bring the edges of the incision together when the muscles are not in contraction.

Now, to obtain this relaxation, deep anaesthesia is required, necessitating large amounts of anaesthetic agents, which are all very toxic substances. The more anaesthetic drug is given, the more difficult will be the patient's recovery and the greater the anaesthetic shock, further aggravating surgical shock.

With a very small dose of curare administered intravenously, the anaesthetist obtained complete muscular relaxation of the whole body: the curare paralysis that Monsieur Lapique had instructed me to show him one day. Curare is only dangerous because it paralyses the respiratory muscles; it is not toxic either to the liver or to the kidneys. The anaesthetists were keen and skilful technicians with curare, and respiratory paralysis was no problem to them, as they always had a respirator, oxygen and even an artificial pulmonary ventilator at hand. And so, thanks to a few milligrams of curare used during operations, they could do away with considerable quantities of ether, chloroform and thiopentone sodium (Pentothal).

The curares used after the Second World War were natural curare extracts, made by the Amazon Indians. Difficult to obtain and to purify, the natural compounds were gradually replaced by synthetic curares made in pharmaceutical laboratories. In the years 1947–8 the Spécia laboratory, affiliated to the Société Rhône-Poulenc, developed a synthetic curare, gallamine triethiodide (Flaxedil), for which the clinical trials had been placed in the hands of Pierre Huguenard, anaesthetist at the Vaugirard Hospital in Paris, who was writing his thesis for a doctorate in medicine on the curares.

An inquisitive doctor, always on the lookout for new methods, Pierre Huguenard, who read all the literature devoted to surgery and anaesthesia, had become interested in articles published by an armed services surgeon on certain effects of the curares that had gone unnoticed. This is how Huguenard came to write to Henri Laborit to ask him for more information.

Laborit, a naval surgeon, was responsible for a surgical outpost based at Sidi Abdalah, near Bizerta in Tunisia. An enlightened doctor who had studied biology, biochemistry and pharmacology (which is rare for surgeons), Laborit had already attracted the attention not only of Pierre Huguenard, but also of surgeons endowed with a medical soul such as the great René Leriche. Laborit had quickly realized the dangers of operative and anaesthetic shock, which robbed surgeons of much operative success; in Tunisia he sought to protect his patients postoperatively by using combinations of medications.

First, he had tried to obtain anaesthesia with the least amount of anaesthetic agent possible, by preparing the patient before the operation, not with a morphine injection alone, but with combinations of medication that potentiated the morphine, and pethidine (a synthetic

opioid). He was thus one of the first to make use of the hypnotic properties of promethazine (Phenergan), which, combined with pethidine
(Dolosal), allowed him to operate with very little anaesthetic. This
research led to his publishing a book entitled *Anaesthesia Facilitated by
Medication Synergies.*

Laborit had also observed that patients well prepared for their operation by good medication combinations did very well postoperatively,
because these medicaments had blocked the sympathetic and parasympathetic nervous systems whose disturbances are responsible not only
for surgical shock, but also for all the 'stress' following physical and psychological trauma.

Huguenard tried to obtain analogous results by perfusing procaine
intravenously in patients undergoing surgery.

Chance, and an administrative requirement, resulted in Laborit being
transferred from Bizerta to Paris, to the Val-de-Grâce Hospital, where a
laboratory was put at his disposal for his research. There, once each
week, he gathered around himself civilian and service researchers, interested and even seduced by his ideas. Pierre Huguenard was one of the
first to participate in these symposia, and a firm friendship soon united
these two doctors who shared the same enthusiasm for research to find a
solution to the 'alarm reaction' of surgical shock.

Laborit's and Huguenard's mixtures

The collaboration between Huguenard and Laborit quickly became
close. The curares were the beginning of it, and the medication combinations suggested by Laborit and tried out by Huguenard made it even
closer.

Each had access to an inexhaustible source of drugs from the hundreds of molecules synthesized by the Rhône-Poulenc–Spécia company. What they wanted was powerfully active substances that put the
famous 'vegetative nervous system' to rest without unduly disturbing
the central nervous system. It was necessary, in some way, to pad the
body rather than 'reinforce' it, so that the surgical trauma would be
cushioned instead of everything being shattered. Already Laborit had
obtained remarkable results with his promethazine–pethidine combination. The protective, hypnotic and antihistaminic properties of promethazine were added to an anti-emetic and analgesic action—by no
means unimportant after an operation. Huguenard and Laborit thought
that it was in the direction of drugs of the same family as promethazine
that they needed to look for more active compounds. The Spécia company had recently marketed a product very closely related to promethazine: Diparcol (diethazine hydrochloride), used in Parkinson's
disease. Laborit, who with his flair had unearthed the product, suggested trying it to Huguenard.

Dip-Dol: Huguenard's first lytic cocktail

Valéry has said that Cleopatra's nose was an everyday event in cosmetic surgery, and that if this pernicious beauty had been made a little uglier, the world would perhaps have been better off.

This was not the case with Madame X who had asked Dr Morel-Fatio to straighten her nose, but who was concerned about the pain she would have to experience. She was a nurse, and had seen in other patients the nose bones being sawn and the nasal septum broken, in similar operations which were performed under local anaesthesia, because one could not put a chloroform or ether mask on the face of a patient undergoing such an operation.

So, on the morning of the operation, even though she wanted it, not only was Madame X anxious, but her distress was accompanied by uncontrollable agitation, making the procedure impossible. It is then that Pierre Huguenard was asked to intervene to calm the patient. There was no question of using the anaesthetic mask, since the operation was on the nose. This is why Huguenard thought of using the mixture he called Dip-Dol (Diparcol–Dolosal), which he gave with atropine and other drugs before surgical operations. However, in general surgery the anaesthesia is continued with ether, chloroform or nitrous oxide, so the patient would be deeply asleep, whereas in the case of Madame X everything happened while she was awake, because she had only local anaesthesia in her nose.

This operation and the account Huguenard gave of it to the Anaesthetic Society in 1950 deserve to be reported, for this constitutes the first description of a state of anxiety, agitation and anguish calmed by a drug synergy without loss of consciousness.

Huguenard, who had watched the behaviour of hundreds of patients after the administration of what he called his 'lytic cocktails', had no hesitation in stating, 'The surprising condition of Madame X after the Dip-Dol injection was, for me, a revelation.'

In a few seconds Madame X's eyes closed, her face became calm, all the agitation disappeared, and her limbs relaxed. But Madame X was not asleep; it was only necessary to ask her a question and she responded with a nod of the head; if pressed, she was capable of speaking. She winced slightly when she had the first procaine injection into her nose, but throughout the operation she remained absolutely calm. With no nausea or feeling of discomfort, she left the operating theatre saying:

'I felt the hammer striking, and the scissor cuts, but as if it was happening to someone else's nose: to me it was indifferent.'

Huguenard picked out the key word: it was 'indifference'. His Dip-Dol cocktail had not only relieved Madame X from a state of agitation and distress, but it had made her feel indifferent to her surroundings, her perceptions, her difficulties and her worries.

At one of the symposia at Val-de-Grâce, organized by Laborit, the case of Madame X was discussed at length, and Huguenard reports that one of the participants, Dr Lassner, no doubt better educated in psychiatry than his colleagues, spoke of pharmacological 'lobotomy', which was an excellent description of what had been achieved. Nevertheless, echoes of the action of the Dip-Dol lytic cocktail never reached the ears of psychiatrists and I do not think it was ever tried in mental illness. One obstacle would present itself in the routine use of Dip-Dol, and this is the presence in the mixture of Dolosal (pethidine): a synthetic morphine-like substance, on the list of narcotic drugs not for routine prescription.

From anaesthetic cocktails to artificial hibernation

With Laborit, who suggested combination formulae, Huguenard prepared his cocktails, inventing increasingly selective and powerful ones. The two workers jointly developed methods that represent the cardinal principles of modern anaesthesia: 'potentiated anaesthesia', 'general anaesthesia without anaesthetic', and even 'wakeful anaesthesia', that is to say, in a wakeful state, since (as in the case of Madame X) it was not necessary for the patient to be asleep in order to be spared from pain.

Huguenard and Laborit pursued the idea, which they tried to inculcate into all anaesthetists and surgeons, that it was better to 'protect the patients undergoing operations with medicinal cocktails, rather than to batter them to death with powerful anaesthetics' [Huguenard].

However, Laborit and Huguenard also observed that their preoperative cocktails put the surgical patient's body to rest—so much so that the body's metabolism was reduced to a minimum, like a hibernating animal. They noticed that in patients treated with these cocktails, if, as sometimes happens, ice-bags are placed on an abdomen, or on a leg prior to amputation for example, the patient's temperature dropped to 35°C or 33°C and that the patients were even more resistant to operative shock. Hence Laborit's and Huguenard's proposal of their method of 'artificial hibernation', involving lowering the temperature of patients undergoing or recovering from serious surgical interventions. To achieve this, six to eight ice bags were used, placed on the abdomen, the folds of the groin, under the arms, on the heart, and on the operation area. In order to stabilize the temperature at 33–35°C, it was necessary to block the vegetative nervous system with the famous lytic cocktails, which contained hypnotics, analgesics, curare and an antihistamine—and obligatorily what Laborit called 'vegetative stabilizers'.

'Barman' Huguenard, who shook the cocktails, asked for stronger and stronger stabilizers. Although satisfied with Phenergan (promethazine) and especially Diparcol (diethazine), which was certainly more powerful, Laborit needed a 'super-stabilizer' to switch the sympathetic system off as completely as possible through an exceptionally powerful action. This is why Laborit went back to the Spécia laboratory to explore the drawers where chemical products kept in reserve or overlooked were lying.

The discovery of chlorpromazine (Largactil)

Promethazine, which Laborit used all the time to begin with, and diethazine hydrochloride, which had given Madame X such perfect indifference in the course of her nose operation, belonged to the same chemical family derived from phenothiazine. It was therefore natural, since one wanted to retain the attributes of diethazine, to chose another product in the same phenothiazine family, and as Laborit asked for the most powerful one, he was given the most toxic.

This was a product which only had a code number (corresponding to the laboratory synthesis book) and two initials: 4560 RP (for Rhône-Poulenc). It had been synthesized by the chemist Paul Charpentier on 11 December 1950, and an initial pharmacology study had been made by Simone Courvoisier.

Compared with promethazine 4560 RP had an additional chlorine atom and it was named chlorpromazine; its commercial name would be Largactil.

Without Laborit, chlorpromazine might perhaps still be in the drawers or on the shelves of a chemical products cupboard at the Spécia laboratory. Why did Courvoisier, or Charpentier, or any other responsible person at Spécia direct this product, rather than any other, to the wisdom of the young surgeon at Val-de-Grâce? We will not seek to know. It is certain that, since his work with Phenergan and Diparcol, Laborit had found that the phenothiazines had undoubted cerebral actions and that Spécia had asked the Rhône-Poulenc research department to pursue the synthesis of phenothiazines.

The rest of the story is very simple. In the hands of 'barman' Huguenard, cocktails of chlorpromazine became so powerful that it took almost nothing to anaesthetize and put a patient into hibernation at 33°C. To combat pain, chlorpromazine potentiates all the analgesics: where three injections of morphine were needed, half of one is enough. The product also counteracts nausea, and is hypnogenic: and it has actions on the heart and blood vessels.

Henri Laborit is young, restless, persuasive; he expresses himself with clarity and logic, and his similes are elegant. He outlines his thoughts and one can see what he is getting at. He is a charmer. René Leriche, the French surgeon of great prestige, has written prefaces for his books. His colleagues, armed services doctors, are envious; his superiors, whose nerves he gets on, champ at the bit since he raises the prestige of military medicine—which it badly needs.

Pierre Huguenard, younger than Laborit, is the unruly child of French anaesthesia; his fieriness, his lack of respect for the bigwigs and mandarins of Parisian surgery make him as many friends as enemies; he is an innovator, in a sphere where more and more surgeons are obliged to recognize the authority of their anaesthetist. For without the anaesthetist, the surgeon could no longer dare to do anything or try anything in a speciality that is entirely composed of risks. And Huguenard says this, and proves it by showing that he resuscitates what the surgeon has had to cut, wound, and sew up again.

Huguenard and Laborit are listened to, read, appreciated, and criticized, but what they do is tried and reproduced by others. Their lytic cocktails and artificial hibernations are breathtaking in their astuteness and their strokes of inspiration. Their technique is followed, and if some difficulty arises, they do not hesitate to personally explain and demonstrate their dexterity to those who have confidence in them.

For chlorpromazine—4560 RP, the product they brought from the oblivion of the chemical stores at Spécia—they are more than enthusiastic; they talk about it in impassioned, lyrical terms, and many people are beginning to try it, a little everywhere, and for no matter what disorder. For beyond their famous cocktails and their premedication to put patients undergoing operations into artificial hibernation, they have been very vague about non-surgical indications. 'Used alone, intravenously, the product does not give rise to any loss of consciousness, or any psychological change, but merely a certain tendency to sleep and a disinterest of the patient for everything going on around him.' For them, 4560 RP is a 'neurovegetative stabilizer'. They recall once more the expression 'pharmacological lobotomy' used by Lassner to characterize the Diparcol–Dolosal cocktail; and they conclude that, '4560 RP (Largactil) is set to extend into many areas including obstetric analgesia and psychiatry.'

To understand what Laborit and Huguenard thought of chlorpromazine, one must refer to the title they gave their paper (with R. Alluaume) in the medical press on 13 February 1952: 'A new neurovegetative stabilizer, 4560 RP.' A psychiatric indication cannot be found in this title, for the neurovegetative system is not (directly at least) implicated in the psychoses. Nevertheless, the possibilities of use in psychiatry was suggested in the paper, and neuropsychiatrists at the Val-de-Grâce Hospital carried out the first trials.

The Val-de-Grâce psychiatric publication on chlorpromazine

Immediately after the paper by Laborit, Huguenard and Alluaume on chlorpromazine, Joseph Hamon, Jean Paraire and Jean Velluz, the psychiatrists at Val-de-Grâce, reported a case of manic agitation treated with chlorpromazine combined with thiopentone sodium and pethidine, and finally cured with electroconvulsive therapy. This was certainly psychiatric treatment with chlorpromazine, but using a method clearly influenced by Huguenard's cocktails. Other authors were subsequently to try the procedure of artificial hibernation in psychiatry, compare chlorpromazine with ganglioplegics, or associate it with the technique of sleep treatment.

The first psychiatrist to recognize the specificity of action of chlorpromazine in psychoses, and show that this product on its own could calm violently agitated patients, and make mentally ill patients indifferent to their delirium, was Pierre Deniker, Professor Jean Delay's assistant, who was in charge of the clinic in the men's department at Sainte-Anne.

Discovery of the neuroleptic* action of chlorpromazine at Sainte-Anne

The mental illness market

'How many do you want for the clinic this morning? One, two? I've got a fine one, here since last night from the Prefecture of Police sick room.'

The Sainte-Anne admissions department supervisor is offering her merchandise to Dr Deniker's house physician. Rather special merchandise, but which has to be distributed as quickly as possible, for the admissions department is refilled every day with ten or fifteen mentally ill patients, collected from inner Paris, who must be passed on straight away because the beds are limited in number. To the admissions department come the 'poor souls', with brains boiling with fury, overwhelmed with anguish, or dead-beat with mental disorder. It is here that the medical certificates are checked, which separate these poor souls from the world they were disturbing or from the dangers to which they were exposing themselves.

The doctor responsible for this department has a considerable role, first verifying the validity of the admission (which was sometimes refused), then providing a diagnosis for each case, and finally transferring the patients to the different departments at Sainte-Anne or the asylums in the nearby area of Paris. By dint of its university hospital status and its responsibility for psychiatric teaching in the Faculty of Medicine, Professor Jean Delay's department had obtained the right from the hospital administrative management to distribute patients sent to it in such a way as to provide a range of patients with sufficiently varied diagnoses, to meet the teaching needs of the students.

And so each morning, before nine o'clock, the house physicians in the clinic, men's and women's departments, went shopping at the admissions department mental illness market.

---

*Everybody knows that *antibiotics* are antimicrobial drugs, intended for treating infections and septicaemias, and that penicillin was the first antibiotic. Similarly *neuroleptics* are drugs for psychoses, intended for treating mental illness, and chlorpromazine (Largactil) was the first neuroleptic.

For several weeks, all who cried, shrieked, gesticulated, spat, all who smashed, threatened, all who had to be tied up, supported, or put in a straitjacket, found a buyer in the closed men's section of the mental illness clinic, of which Dr Pierre Deniker was the departmental head.

As a rule, this category of patient was not particularly welcome, because of the disturbances created in the wards, where the tumult and agitation were propagated by contagion. It was not much of a gift when one received a maniacal patient who for weeks would shriek, and injure other patients; who had to be put in a straitjacket, and even tied to the bed with straps, and who had with difficulty to be made to eat, and to be kept clean.

Now, for some time, to the head admissions doctor's satisfaction, all the manic patient provision was running along smoothly: there was no longer any problem in distributing this undesirable merchandise. Deniker took it all.

As this strange appetite for agitated, confused, acutely delirious people was being marvelled at, the house physician who came shopping said mysteriously:

'We've found a trick that works.'

Yes, it worked, all right. Indeed, it worked very well. It had worked almost at once. First, however, it had been necessary to carry out trials, and above all, to observe and to persevere, then be specific about a method that was going to revolutionize first the therapy of excitation and manic agitation, then the delirium of the major psychoses.

The calm after the storm

I was Pierre Deniker's house physician in 1949. We were both clinic chiefs in 1950–1, he in the men's department (confined, insane people), and I in the free department (voluntary in-patients), which I left in the autumn of 1951 to become Director of the Biology Laboratory, which was a few tens of metres from the patients' wards. As my research dealt essentially with the analysis of in-patient cases, each morning I spent several hours with my colleagues in the department, and took part in daily ward rounds and in therapies the results of which I checked in the laboratory.

Pierre Deniker, like Pierre Pichot (Jean Delay's other assistant) and myself, was firmly dedicated to biological and therapeutic psychiatry. This was the choice Jean Delay had made for the orientation of his teaching and the instructions given to his collaborators. This did not prevent him from welcoming all psychotherapies, analytical or otherwise, which were widely represented in his department, including Jacques Lacan, who organized his seminars there.

Whereas the more analytical and speculative mind of Pierre Pichot had taken him in the direction of psychometric measurements and evaluations, Pierre Deniker and I were above all attracted by therapeutics and the psychiatric pharmacology that was little by little taking shape, and for which we had cleared the overgrown terrain.

Deniker had developed therapy with dinitriles; for my own part I had studied the anti-alcoholic action of Antabuse, developed some new anti-epileptics, and demonstrated the absence of any addictive tendency with pholcodine, which became one of the most widely used antitussives.

My studies on curare and relaxation by infracurarization had familiarized me with the work of Laborit, and I had met Huguenard at the Society of Anaesthesia, where I had presented papers on new curarizants and local anaesthetic agents, but in the course of these meetings we had never spoken about the calming actions of lytic cocktails and artificial hibernation. It was from his surgeon brother-in-law that Pierre Deniker learnt of Laborit's and Huguenard's experiments in hibernation with chlorpromazine.

'The patients are overcome, calm, and passive under hibernation; you can do what you like with them. Why not try it for agitated mental patients?'

Pierre Deniker, who was unacquainted with Laborit and Huguenard, asked the Spécia laboratory directly for samples of chlorpromazine. Dr Beal, in charge of clinical trials at Spécia, sent him some ampoules and a small Roneotyped note on the pharmacology (very brief) of the product and on the technique of hibernation. I remember seeing the first patients treated with chlorpromazine injections, for I often went from my laboratory into the patients' wards to take blood samples and carry out biological analyses.

Stretched out on their beds, calm and drowsy, or with a fixed gaze, lost in a limitless distance, these patients had been set free from their strait-waistcoats and hemp straitjackets. Sometimes, bags of tepid water slid from their sheets, for in the early days of the treatment, which followed, for good or bad, the principles of hibernation, at the same time as chlorpromazine was administered, ice packs were placed on the patients' bodies. This useless refrigeration soon had to be given up; firstly because keeping ice packs on an agitated body required extraordinary skill and perseverance, and secondly because the pharmacy service, which provided the ice, declared it could not cope with the demand.

'Anyway, it doesn't achieve anything,' said the nurses, 'the injections are enough.'

This was immediately understood by Deniker, who was the first to grasp the importance of the sedation obtained with chlorpromazine. He analysed the behaviour of the agitated, shrieking, gesticulating patient who soon after the injection calmed down and lay peacefully on the bed. This was not the irresistible sleep produced by a hypnotic or even promethazine, but a reduction in alertness, which did not prevent the patient from responding to questions. More striking still, the physical calmness produced by the medication was accompanied by psychological sedation; the insults, sarcasms, and outrageous and absurd words lessened in intensity, and little by little died away.

Strangely, this return to calm was accompanied by a lessening in mental confusion and a re-establishment of normal thought processes. Delirious patients admitted to the department a short time previously, who could not give the day, the month or even the year of their hospitalization, or know where they were or the circumstances that had led to their arrival at the hospital, regained their orientation, remembered the beginning of their illness, and began to discuss their case.

All this went on in peace and serenity. The hemp waistcoats were put back in the cupboards, and the hydrotherapy pools were only used for personal washing. In the corridors of Deniker's department one no longer passed patients in shirts walking with their straitjackets open with straps undone on the way to the toilets, but patients dressed in heavy blue cloth, strolling decently and quietly as far as the rest room. And if the fury and violence had given way to calmness and peace, the most evident sign of this extraordinary therapeutic result could be appreciated even from the outside of the building of the men's clinic—there was *silence*.

I can no longer remember who it was who said that the results obtained with chlorpromazine could be measured in the psychiatric hospitals in decibels (units of sound intensity) recorded before and after the introduction of this drug. In fact, Deniker's department was a small island of silence in Sainte-Anne, where the cries of rage of the mentally ill patients often disturbed people living in the neighbouring roads.

Chlorpromazine in strong doses

The results obtained by Deniker were the consequence of close clinical observation of patients treated with chlorpromazine and an analysis of the first reactions obtained with strong doses of the product.

For Laborit and Huguenard had used chlorpromazine extensively, but in small doses and in association with other narcotics (pethidine, promethazine, etc.), which had partly concealed the specific action of the product from them.

Deniker, who like all psychiatrists could not base a therapy on the daily prescription of a drug capable of inducing addiction, had administered chlorpromazine on its own, without mixing it with opioids. This made it easier to analyse and characterize the specific essential action of the product, no longer masked by other hypnotic derivatives. Deniker also noticed that the doses of chlorpromazine given by Laborit and Huguenard were insufficient when the product was given on its own, and it was to his credit that he dared to give four or six times as much of the product in order to obtain effective results.

These doses, which were perfectly well tolerated by the patients, enabled the outstanding psychosedative properties of the new drug, only glimpsed by previous experimenters, to be revealed.

Jean Delay, informed by Deniker of the results obtained, immediately became interested in chlorpromazine, but before reporting the observations gathered to scientific societies, he wanted a larger number of cases of cure, and recommended the collection into Deniker's department of all patients presenting with states of excitation, agitation, and mental confusion arriving at the admissions department at Sainte-Anne.

From May until July 1952 Delay and Deniker were thus able to present six scientific papers covering more than forty observations on psychoses and underlining the importance of 'continuous and prolonged' treatment with chlorpromazine in states of manic agitation and acute psychoses.

A few other psychiatrists had also used chlorpromazine, but only in association with other products, either following the hibernation technique or sleep treatment, or to potentiate the barbiturates, which as a result concealed the product's own action and its possibilities from them. The originality of Deniker's research was to have used chlorpromazine in strong doses, alone, without hibernation and without sleep treatment.

The first mental illness medication

It must not be thought that what is today an obvious fact was accepted immediately by everybody. We were a small group, astonished, surprised, and fired with enthusiasm by these results. In my own laboratory I used chlorpromazine to carry out extraordinary animal experiments, about which I will speak later, which allowed characterization of the properties of this new class of drug, called *neuroleptics*. This term, accepted in France and generally in Europe, was not unanimously accepted everywhere in the world, especially in the USA. This is at once an injustice and a prejudiced reaction which takes no account of the French discovery or of the perfect neological construction of the word. Jean Delay, in coining the word 'neuroleptic' to characterize the action of chlorpromazine, had followed precisely the phonetic and semantic laws of etymology. Chlorpromazine was a neuroleptic drug, he said, because 'this substance which permeates the body of the patient for whom it is prescribed, attaches itself to the nervous system, depressing it selectively, settling the excited mind.'

Regardless of definitions, neologisms and clinical descriptions, the discovery was there, precise, stunning and clear: *for the first time a drug cured major mental disorders, without relying upon sleep, hydrotherapy, or electric or insulin shock.* Calming agitation, soothing delirium, it achieved the long-awaited objective of all psychiatrists: to reduce as quickly as possible all signs of mental illness and to restore a mental state that would make a good quality of family and social reintegration possible.

The question of time was important. Before the use of chlorpromazine, mentally ill patients often stayed for months or even years in asylums or psychiatric clinics. With this drug, a calmed patient could be free of delirium within a few days, and leave the hospital within a few weeks. Better still, the new drug showed other therapeutic properties; clearing a way into the tormented mind, it did not solely calm excitation and the ramblings of delirium, it also freed the inhibitions of the person struck down by passivity, inaction and autism, restoring contact with a world which had been shut off.

The curing of Philippe Burg

Sophie Burg had been a dresser for many years in one of our greatest Parisian theatres, and when she retired, at the reception organized in her honour, she brought a tall, blond young man whom she introduced as her son. Everybody was surprised, for Mlle Sophie had never spoken of him throughout her professional life. When asked what her son was doing, she answered with pride:

'He wants to be an archaeologist; he is at the École du Louvre.'

Philippe Burg had been brought up at his mother's sister's home at Châteauroux; he had been educated at the Alphonse XIII College, and after his baccalauréat, he had gone up to Paris for further studies on the history of art and archaeology. He lived with his mother in the rue de Vaugirard, in a small apartment in an old building near the rue de Rennes. Sophie Burg had managed to obtain the additional use of a former maid's room, on the top floor, under the roof, where she had furnished a study for Philippe with a divan where he slept. The boy was pleasant, quiet, and hard-working. He passed his examinations and competitions successfully, and he had a few friends whom he never introduced to his mother, to whom he seldom spoke.

'It was me who made all the conversation,' said Sophie, 'but he always answered when I asked him questions. I knew nothing about Patricia when she came to see me.'

Patricia L was also at the École du Louvre; she was a young woman from Marseilles, with a delightful accent, who appeared embarrassed to be telling this story to Sophie Burg.

'You must understand, Madame. I thought he had spoken to you about it a long time ago: we were to have been married by now, in the spring, but he told me he would prefer to postpone the date till the autumn, when you would be retired. I wanted to meet you, and get to know you, but he always put the meeting off until later. And then when this happened, and I told him I was pregnant, he told me he would bring me to your home the next day; now I have not seen him again for three days. He is not coming to the course any more, so I decided to come to see you.'

Sophie Burg went pale. She, too, had not seen Philippe for two days. He told her that he was going to Chartres to attend a seminar on religious sculpture. Patricia had never heard of this seminar.

The two women looked for Philippe in Paris, notified his disappearance at the nearest police station and at the Prefecture of Police, and awaited news with anguish. And then one day a message boy on a bicycle, an urgent message; the Commissariat again, the journey in the special Infirmary taxi from the quai de Gesvres to the rue Cabanis, the great entrance at Sainte-Anne.

'Your son has been found again, Madame, at the Guimet museum, in the Tibetan antiquities room, in front of the Buddha Mahayana: he had taken off all his clothes and was squatting in the lotus position, with a bell in his hand.'

The Guimet museum is little frequented: the rooms are dark and the guardian, dozing on his chair, had not noticed the man undressing himself in front of the Buddha.

'As for me, you know, doctor,' said Sophie Burg, 'I did not know Philippe very well. I so seldom saw him. When the show finished in Paris, I often went on tour with the set. My sister told me he was quiet and affectionate; perhaps too solitary. When he came to Paris, it was a great joy to have him near me. I did not notice anything abnormal.'

Sophie Burg began a long tale of suffering: this son she had borne when very young, by a comedian who never wanted to acknowledge him, this boy brought up far away from her by her sister; she now no longer wanted to leave him. She needed him back, she would come for him; it would turn out to be not so bad as it looked. As Philippe remained calm and appeared to be getting on better, he was returned to his mother. Meantime, Patricia had an abortion and broke off all relations with the Burgs. Philippe did not go back to the École du Louvre. In spite of all his mother's efforts, he little by little sank into the maze of his fuzzy thoughts: extreme nonchalance, hours of silent solitude on his bed. Sophie made him go out for a daily walk in the Luxembourg gardens.

And then, one winter evening, during the night, in Sophie's house— cries and shrieks, flames in Philippe's attic room. He was cold and he set fire to his books. He was successfully removed from the fire, half-asphyxiated and badly burnt.

Back again at Sainte-Anne, weekly visits by Sophie Burg whom Philippe no longer recognized. This time the world had closed for him, just as he had shut himself off from all social obligations and emotional contacts. With his mother's agreement he was given a series of six, then twelve, then up to thirty insulin comas, with no improvement, without the smallest sign that a puff of spirit and emotion persisted in this still-living corpse. His body became very big after the Sakel treatments. Philippe was a mass of flesh, a mountain of fat, dragging himself from bed to canteen bench, from canteen bench to the exercise yard, indifferent to everything; to the world, to himself; drawn only by the meals which give some rhythm to the days.

He had been in this state for three years when I met him. Arriving as the new clinic head in the department, I had been given his notes, where

I read what I have recounted above. I had also greeted his mother, always more weighed down, always thinner, dressed in black, who wanted to know from the new doctor who was to have the care of her son whether by any chance there was any new treatment. No more than my colleagues could I remove Philippe's possibly still living soul from the nets in which it was caught. At Sophie Burg's pressing request, I carried out one final Sakel treatment, which was the last he underwent.

The nurse who supervised comas said to me, 'It took nearly a litre of glucose to wake him up, and he is taking a kilo every day.'

The only action he carried out quickly was a rapid movement of his right forearm and hand to catch flies. He pulled off their wings and watched them wandering on his enormous palm, or else put them on his bed sheet which he folded to make obstacles.

At the end of my clinic year, I changed departments and did not see Philippe again any more. It was a nurse who spoke to me about him two years later.

Following the old custom of therapeutic psychiatrists who try things 'to see', Philippe was given some chlorpromazine to take. And besides, Sophie Burg had undoubtedly heard the miracle drug spoken about; she insisted that it should be given to her son, even though his case was not an ideal indication. What happened in his enormous carcass? A stir, a tidal wave caused three words to spring to Philippe's mute lips, 'Sophie's bad luck.'

He repeated them twice more during the day, at mealtimes, 'Sophie's bad luck. Sophie's bad luck.'

Then the doses were increased. Philippe weighed 120 kilos; he was given progressively up to 600 mg of chlorpromazine daily. This was a long way from Laborit and Huguenard's cocktails of 50–100 mg. Saturation of the giant with the drug produced a strange result. For a long time he could be seen to be fighting against a lethargy which was little by little overcoming him. He walked slowly, heavily, lengthening his pace, arms held away from his trunk; sometimes he turned back, as if he had been called; having succeeded in remaining standing up, leaning against one of the plane trees in the nearby covered walking area, he let himself slide to the ground. Two male nurses lifted him up and helped him to his bed, where he stretched himself out. He did not sleep but lay with his eyes closed, muttering incomprehensible sentences, or else with his eyes wide open, staring at the ceiling, he outlined with his finger things that were visible to him alone.

The chlorpromazine mobilized currents, emotional and affective drives, in the innermost recesses of his enormous carcass; as the passage of a dragnet would have done at the bottom of a muddy swamp.

What was suffocated, dulled and exhausted in the network of his psychosis was shaken up by the dragnet and was now rushing towards the surface of his consciousness; but there, again, there was an obstacle, for it had to cross contrary currents and eddies—a swirling maelstrom that had formed years ago; an impassable barrier to the restoration of basic instincts, feelings, emotions and affective memories.

Philippe tossed restlessly on his bed, but without violence or impulsive movements. In the jerks of emotion that had troubled him he recalled words, scrap of sentences, again badly put together.

'The runes are leaving the stones . . .'

He had to be made to repeat this phrase several times. The nurses had written it down in the care book. At first they had written 'ruins'—'The ruins are leaving the stones'—and then corrected this later, because Philippe had got up and gone over to the dormitory wall where, with the tips of his fingers, he outlined signs, murmuring all the time, 'The runes are leaving the stones.'

A nurse had asked him: 'What ruins?'

He turned round angrily, screaming, 'Runes! Runes!'

It was discovered that before his first admission, he was working on a thesis about old Scandinavian texts written in runic characters. One of his former teachers said that some runic texts only existed engraved on stones and that Philippe, to study them, took tracings of them on large sheets of paper.

For a few weeks, he seemed to be upset by jolts of recalled consciousness, which were split up and scattered; then once more, despite the chlorpromazine that he was given every day, he relapsed into lifeless apathy. And then one Thursday, after family visiting, the head nurse saw Sophie Burg, still dressed in black, come into his office and rush up to him.

'Monsieur Thomas! Monsieur Thomas! He has spoken to me. He called me mother. Mother!'

Sophie Burg cried and laughed; emotion gripped her throat and her heart was beating so forcibly that she had to sit down for a moment behind the oak desk, on Thomas's cane chair, who was himself so moved that he forgot to finish rolling his cigarette, and the tobacco fell out from the paper.

Castin, the secretary of the department, told me what happened.

'If you had seen the scene, sir. There she was, quite wild; it was as if her son had been brought back to life for her. She wanted to kiss us. The next Sunday she brought us a bottle of sparkling Vouvray; I will always remember the brand: 'le Peu de la Mauriette'. We wanted to drink it with her, but she declined, wine made her head spin, she had not drunk any for a long time.'

And so, little by little, Philippe emerged from an indefinable mist, from a colourless, vaporous world; at first unsteady, his mind shaken by a wave that had come to shatter his inertia, he came out of the straitjacket that had imprisoned him. His speech, indistinct and confused, became clearer, and his uneasy jolting gait became steadier. The formation and linking-up of ideas only came back slowly and in a partial way, but a few days' home leave could be considered.

It was Castin again who told me about this first outing.

'You understand: the problem: it was the clothes. Philippe had got so fat that all the garments his mother had kept for him for seven years were unwearable. But she didn't want to take him out in the blue drape hospital uniform. So it was fixed up. Sophie Burg bought a length of cloth, and Pinton, the asylum tailor, took his measurements and made him a suit. When she wanted to pay him, he told her it was the hospital's gift.'

She came to fetch him one Sunday morning in September. They left the hospital on foot. She had said:

'The rue de Rennes is not far, and we'll do it walking.'

And he, in his fine new coat, had wanted to take his mother's arm, like a child being led. But very soon, after the small privet hedge which marked the entrance to the department, Sophie Burg had switched the roles. Unhesitatingly, she had pushed her son's arm away, and it was now hers which rested on Philippe's arm, so that when they crossed the Sainte-Anne gateway, it looked as though it was he who was taking his mother out from the hospital.

They went for lunch at the Closerie des Lilas, then walked around the Luxembourg gardens. She hesitated to take him to her home, but decided to do so because he looked tired. He lay down on his bed, and for an hour she watched him doze.

She rediscovered, with this adult whose brain was barely awakening from a long sleep, feelings and attitudes which she had not known when her sister had brought up her son in her place.

In the evening she took him back to the hospital. Everything had gone well. His fine new suit was put away until the next home leave.

Perfecting the neuroleptics

The neuroleptic action of chlorpromazine was thus not only a powerful and selective calming effect, which stopped the patient from crying out and becoming agitated, without inducing sleep; it was also a radical action which dissolved delirium and hallucinations, and roused the patient from the torpor and prostration resulting from the psychosis.

Psychiatrists learnt over time to distinguish the two actions, the sedative, calming action and the disinhibiting action, which freed the patient from mental paralysis. The well-differentiated characteristics of these two actions subsequently led to the introduction of neuroleptic drugs that were predominantly sedative for agitated states, or predominantly disinhibiting for delirium and hallucinatory psychoses.

In this way another step forward was taken a few years later, when the Belgian Paul Jansen introduced haloperidol (Haldol), which proved a powerful neuroleptic in psychoses with hallucinations, for which the drug has an almost specific action. Subsequently, this therapy was further refined by the manufacture of long-acting or 'retard' neuroleptics. This is because patients with chronic psychoses require neuroleptic medication on a long-term basis. After the improvement obtained in the hospital or clinic, when the patient returns home it is difficult to maintain the treatment, either because it is thought unnecessary when everything seems to be going well, or because it is considered dangerous to go on taking a drug permanently. However, it is important to understand that while treatment with neuroleptics has a curative action in acute psychoses, it only has a suspensory action in most chronic psychoses, notably in schizophrenia: a few days or weeks after prematurely stopping the medication, the delirium returns and a further hospital admission is necessary.

Neuroleptics with a prolonged action have been developed; a single intramuscular injection of one of these 'retard' neuroleptics can be enough for a therapeutic effect lasting for three or even four weeks. The advantages of these preparations are many. Treatment with the drug can be controlled by a general practitioner; administration of the medication is simplified, and the total number of doses is reduced, diminishing the risks of long-term toxicity.

The manufacture in the future of drugs with an even longer duration action can be envisaged, but this leads to other considerations of the moral kind, which we shall discuss further.

The French reaction

How was the discovery of the neuroleptic action of chlorpromazine perceived and welcomed in France?

The results obtained were surprising, and unexpected: it became necessary to explain, demonstrate and convince. What is now generally accepted, what is 'self-evident' for young psychiatrists today, was not immediately accepted by those of the 1950s. There were immediate followers, with enquiring minds, who set up trials and were more or less rapidly convinced. Among these, a Lyons school was formed, which was enthusiastic from the start.

There were also those who, willingly or not, lost their way along blind alleys. Thus some, deliberately, wanted to carry out artificial hibernation, following Huguenard and Laborit; this was useless, dangerous and superfluous, and it masked the true action of chlorpromazine. Others wanted to put neuroleptic treatment with chlorpromazine into the same category as a ganglioplegic treatment, and compared it with this type of drug, taking no account of the pharmacological action of the product. Hamon, Paraire and Velluz, who had first spoken about chlorpromazine, persisted in associating it with the hypnotics, thus showing that they had not made use of its specific action. Finally, others regarded the method as a new technique for sleep treatment, which was the most serious error.

In spite of these minor setbacks, Delay and Deniker gathered observations and published their results, insisting on the necessity of prolonging treatment in strong doses taken continuously. Therapeutic successes followed in large numbers, and demands for the drug at the Spécia laboratory multiplied, so they decided to market the product.

At first Spécia mainly saw a commercial outlet in the indications recommended by Laborit and Huguenard, that is to say essentially in anaesthesia, and also as a drug likely to be used with other drugs to reinforce their action. It is for these reasons that the trade name 'Largactil' was chosen, derived from the words 'large action'. It is evident that this term took no account of the neuroleptic action of the product and its major application in the treatment of mental illness.

Spécia was initially surprised at the applications of chlorpromazine in psychiatry, but quickly realized the commercial value of this outlet. Information briefings were organized in various university centres in Europe. Deniker travelled widely describing the method he had introduced. Foreign doctors came to Paris, to Sainte-Anne, to learn the details of the technique. The USA alone, with their customary reserve concerning anything going on in Europe, seemed to take little interest, especially as it concerned psychiatry, which, in their country, was in the hands of psychoanalysts. A few interested doctors, however, came to Sainte-Anne, such as Herman Denber of New York.

If Mohammed would not go to the mountain, the chlorpromazine had to go to the USA. Pierre Deniker and Henri Laborit met in the aeroplane that took them to the USA and Canada, where they made a tour of conferences to speak, respectively, about the use of chlorpromazine in psychiatry and in surgery. The first report of the action of chlorpromazine on the American continent was by the Canadian, Heinz Lehmann, from Montreal, but only at the beginning of 1954. It was difficult to establish the drug in the USA, which did not accept the name Largactil, and changed it to Thorazine.

However, an American was going to find a neuroleptic himself, a drug acting on psychoses.

Rauwolfia, reserpine, and Nathan S. Kline

Rauwolfia serpentina is the rather complicated name of a plant that, principally in India, has long been used to treat numerous illnesses. It is a small shrub with red flowers, about fifty centimetres in height, whose roots have an undulating shape reminiscent of the body of a snake, from which the various names of 'serpentine' and '*sorpa-gandha*' (which repels snakes) were given to the plant to evoke its use against snake bites. But the plant also had other names in Hindi, such as *chabdra* (moon) and *pagla-ka-dawa* (fool's herb), for it was also used as a remedy for lunatics and madmen.

Unknown in Europe until the beginning of the seventeenth century, the plant was first described by the French botanist Plumier, who called it

Rauwolfia after the German doctor and botanist Leonard Rauwolf, who had studied oriental medicinal plants in 1574.

It was only in 1930 that fresh interest was taken in the medicinal properties of *Rauwolfia*, when two Indians, S. Siddiqui and R. Siddiqui, isolated five alkaloids from the plant, and two other Indian doctors, Ganneth Sen and Katrick Bose, described the use of *Rauwolfia* in the treatment of hypertension. Subsequently, in Europe, total extracts of the plant were prepared, and in Switzerland the Ciba laboratories in Basle succeeded in isolating the active alkaloid, reserpine, which they successfully synthesized and sold under the name of Serpasil.

All the *Rauwolfia*-based products were very active in hypertension and were prescribed for a great number of patients throughout the world. The credit of discovering the neuroleptic action of *Rauwolfia* belongs to the American psychiatrist Nathan S. Kline.

On several occasions, in his department at Rockland State Hospital in New York State, he had looked after patients with depression, some of whom had even made suicide attempts. Now, these patients were also being treated with *Rauwolfia* extracts or reserpine for arterial hypertension. Kline drew a link between the depression developing in his patients and the treatment of their hypertension, and thought that the administration of *Rauwolfia* was responsible for their depression. To convince himself, he gave agitated patients increasing doses of *Rauwolfia*, and succeeded in calming them. Similarly, doses of reserpine, ten to twenty times greater than those used to treat hypertension, gave remarkable results in some acute and chronic psychoses.

Kline announced his first observations on psychoses treated with *Rauwolfia* at the New York Academy of Sciences on 30 April 1954; that is to say, about two years after Delay's and Deniker's publication regarding chlorpromazine. The reception for the treatment proposed by Kline was made more favourable by the prior discovery of chlorpromazine, for the fact that medication could be effective in the psychoses had already been established. The use of reserpine, more manageable than *Rauwolfia* extracts, quickly became widespread, but although active, this drug was supplanted by other more effective neuroleptics, and in practice neither *Rauwolfia* nor reserpine are now used to treat psychoses.

The first Paris Colloquium on the neuroleptics: 20–22 October 1955

The game of congresses, colloquia, symposia and seminars is governed by precise rules, and is a production where everyone has a part to play. Usually people speak in order to listen to themselves, to discuss, or to introduce counter-arguments. The curious come as witnesses, to judge, to count the points in the course of the oratorical jousts, and to draw conclusions. It must be said that sometimes useful clarifications, if not knowledge, spring from these discussions.

At the 1950 World Psychiatry Congress, discussion had been lively on shock therapies; at the colloquium on neuroleptics organized at Sainte-Anne in 1955 the theme was the new chemical therapeutics, and there was complete agreement amongst all the participants: chlorpromazine and reserpine were recognized as major discoveries in the treatment of mental illness. On the rostrum of the great amphitheatre in Jean Delay's department, French and foreign psychiatrists followed one another, all proclaiming the quality of the results obtained with these new drugs. Hans Hoff from Vienna, Aksel from Istanbul, Felix Labarth from Basle, Linford Rees from London, Sarro from Barcelona, Manfred Bleuler from Zürich, and Willy Mayer-Gross from Birmingham came to say that this was the first time in the history of psychiatry that a drug gave such concordant results (they were speaking particularly of chlorpromazine). There were only two Americans at this reunion, Winfred from Washington and Denber from New York. They, too, were affirmative. Denber had succeeded in showing that even the experimental psychoses were susceptible to chlorpromazine. He had successfully dissipated mescaline hallucinations with an injection of fifty milligrams of chlorpromazine.

Henri Ey, who also took part in this colloquium, described what he called the 'hallucinolytic' properties of chlorpromazine.

Not without humour, the Dutchman H. C. Rümke suggested that if Freud had been present, perhaps he would have been happy to hear so many psychiatrists convinced of the effect of a drug in mental illness: and he quoted Van Ophuyzen, who had reported this sentence from the celebrated Austrian psychoanalyst: 'You know, I am firmly convinced that one day all these mental troubles, which we try to understand through psychoanalysis, will be treated by means of hormones or similar substances, and I will be glad if this is in the near future.' Evidently, Freud thought of hormones because his pathogenic conceptions were tied to sexual and libido problems; but he had never been an adversary of drugs.

The neuroleptics and the psychoanalysts

The attitude of psychotherapeutic psychiatrists faced with the results obtained with the neuroleptics had been quite strange. Certainly, the indications for a psychoanalytically inspired psychotherapy were different from those for chemotherapy with neuroleptics, but some ardent supporters of psychotherapy could not refrain from looking enviously at the speed of some of the results obtained with drugs, compared with the slowness of improvement achieved by other means. Moreover, the use of drugs, particularly the neuroleptics, was always a problem for psychoanalysts. For little secrets on the couch, the analysis of what was said, the transference of affect, or the evolution through time of concepts allowed to settle in the course of the sessions, was a poor match for taking tablets, the action of which was felt immediately.

Some found clever ways of avoiding losing face. Thus one of these psychoanalysts, whose talent and competence it is my duty to recognize, said to his patients:

'It would be good for some of the symptoms you show [nervousness, insomnia, irritation, anxiety, distress] to have them treated by a colleague who will prescribe a few pills.'

Beforehand, the colleague in question was warned to prescribe the chosen drug in precise conditions studied in advance.

'You understand,' this psychoanalyst said to me, 'this way I do not compromise myself, and thanks to you, I remain effective.'

I often went along with this merry-go-round, which, I must maintain, had only the interests of the patient (who was thus perfectly safeguarded) as its objective.

Prelude to an interlude

Beside the psychoanalysts who retained their methods but remained open to psychopharmacological discoveries, there were also the hard core who refused to compromise themselves with anything that was not their own view. I will not throw any stones at them, for the freedom of their practice was the more to be respected since psychotherapy is—and will remain—one of the therapeutic methods that are essential in the treatment of mental illness. Far be it from me to claim that chemotherapy is the panacea for neuroses and psychoses; I merely wish to underline the sectarianism of those who deny its place in the therapy of these illnesses.

They were many who went with disdain through this period of the discovery of the neuroleptics without any concern for what it brought to a discipline in which they had chosen to trace their path in the labyrinths of the subconscious, only to come out from it again through narrow doors.

I have said that Henri Ey had quickly opened his department to chemotherapy with neuroleptics. He did it in full agreement with his concept of the pathogenesis of the psychoses. For identical reasons, Jacques Lacan rightly took no interest in these new therapies, and my intention should not be to put him in the picture in this chapter where he has nothing to do; but, having spoken of him earlier when I had known him competing in oratory skills with Henri Ey, in calculated jousts, still accessible to the comprehension of the young pupil that I was, I could not resist the urge to give an account of one of my last meetings with the master of the Freudian school in Paris.

From neuroleptics to a Lacan seminar

I greatly admired Lacan, because his intelligence fitted him like a glove. There are people who do not wear theirs well; it is generally not their fault, but they are responsible, in spite of everything, for their intelligence, just as one is for one's nose or the coat one has chosen for oneself.

It was because I had been attracted by Lacan's intelligence, from the time of the meetings at Bonneval, that I wanted to see what remained of it after the discovery of the neuroleptics. It might be said that this is beside the point, but let us have a closer look. For me, it was a pilgrimage to shrines of disappointed love affairs. I have spoken of my feelings of helplessness in the therapeutic desert in which I began my career in psychiatry; before turning towards psychopharmacology, my 'high spots', as you might say, had been those Wednesday teaching sessions with Henri Ey, and the colloquia and discussions with Lacan which I subsequently enjoyed reading. This is why in the hurly-burly of pragmatic therapeutics, the full-time job in research rich in promise and fruitful discoveries, in the middle of my neurochemical work on the biochemical concept of psychosis, in this beginning of a chemotherapy of mental illness that was building up every day, I wanted to see and hear what had become of the 'word', what was being constructed from his pyramids of verbiage. I wanted to compare. Not to judge, for my decision was already made, but to make sure of my reason or what I had required of it. This is why I attended the show that I describe here as an interlude.

The laboratory where I did my experiments and where I checked the action of the neuroleptics was a few steps from the department to which I went every morning. I never went into the wards without saying 'hello' to the nurse in charge, Madame Cothias. Her office was a meeting place where house physicians, doctors and clinic heads came to chat before the patient presentations or teaching sessions. Sometimes I met Jacques Lacan there, on the days he held his seminars.

I had heard much about these seminars, of their mixed audiences, the show the master put on, and of their success. I told him I would like to come one day to one of his talks.

'Entry is free whenever you wish.'

I explained about my work, the fixed timetable, the experiments that required checking just at the time of his lecture, which began around midday and ended in the afternoon. Then one day, I managed to be free.

In the head nurse's office, Lacan was waiting for the room to fill up. To try to get my bearings in his presentation, I asked him on the off chance what he was going to talk about.

'You'll soon see,' he answered, 'But you'd better move now if you want a seat.'

Indeed, the amphitheatre was almost full. There were students from all disciplines, famous comedians, priests, socialites, psychiatrists of course, and individuals whose appearance and behaviour gave away the reasons for their presence.

The stenotypist was sitting ready at a small table on the platform. The large blackboard was carefully cleaned, and the box of chalks placed at one end of the big table covered with green cloth. At about midday, Jacques Lacan made his entrance into the room. He slowly descended the steps from the door to the bottom of the room, elbowing his way through the audience already seated on the steps, and he stepped on to the platform.

With his eyes highlighted with small gold-rimmed spectacles, crew-cut grey hair, bow tie neatly positioned on the shirt collar, and jacket lapels of broad cut, it was Jacques Lacan's duty to look good for his audience, and so he did.

Standing facing his audience, he first closed his eyes, then opened them slowly as if he was coming out of a deep sleep. At first almost surprised at his gathering, he looked away from it, took a few steps to the right, then to the left, stretched out an arm in front as if to make a shade, appeared to talk to himself, and suddenly seemed to discover his stenotypist toward whom he turned. He said a few words in her ear, then appeared to be hunting in his pockets for something mislaid; he eventually took out a few pieces of paper which he smoothed flat on a corner of the big green-covered table; he appeared to examine them to read a few notes; then, still standing in the middle of the platform and after putting his arm out in front once more, he began his address.

From this single Lacan spectacle at which I was present, I cannot make any general analysis, but I believe in a certain permanence of the fame of the individual. I enjoy recounting the private conversation I had with him that day. For he was in front of me, as if it was just the two of us there together, to exchange confidences.

After referring briefly to what he had said at the previous lecture, he began to talk, slowly at first, then in an increasingly animated way, walking backwards and forwards. Sometimes he wrote a sentence or a proper name, usually illegible, on the blackboard, or else drew something indecipherable, which he came back to explain, adding supplementary graffiti, punctuated with blows struck with the chalk on the black wood.

The tone, the attraction, and the linking of the sentences was magnificent, and the charm worked little by little on the whole audience, who were first seduced, then in ecstasy, and finally bewitched by the play of a most magic style, a superb phraseology, and by the extraordinary paradox of an actor who played a major part while speaking a phantom text. For Lacan's sentences had the prodigious quality of being perfectly constructed, with all the logical constituents of speech, but with so many ramblings and antinomies, that comprehension was lost between the subject and the complement, the verb and the object. Faced with the impossibility of understanding any of the verbiage, I felt struck with agnosia, and verbal deafness, understanding nothing of what the speaker said, and all the more anguished to see that the audience was hanging on his lips.

This went on for two hours, in the course of which, first irritated, then amused, and finally fascinated by the spectacle, I gave way to looking at all these people who were taking notes, certainly unfamiliar with this lecture. But after all, was this not the much sought-after object of the exercise? I was also fascinated by the tone the orator adopted, and which at times rose in sarcasm or dropped into lament; in turn cheerful, making fun of people, vehement, he played in all registers and employed every nuance. But the eyes were also working through the golden glasses; their power over these fanatics was as real as the actor's dialogue and acting.

So I confess to have grasped nothing logical in this conference, but so that nobody puts this portrait and account down to an invention made up from scattered reports, I am going to detail a point in the talk that Lacan gave that day and that surely the listeners, and perhaps even the speaker himself, might remember if by any chance they ever read this.

It was a question of hedgehogs. How do they come into this story involving trouble, with the speaker's emotive language delivered in such impassioned style?

'The false question was love. What should he believe? Look at the hedgehog! Problem! Two hedgehogs. Two problems. And love! The solution. Think of the soft belly, of the spikes on the back. Flattened in normal times, these spikes, but susceptible to erection. And the erection, the other one, the true one, that of mating! How will they do it? Eh? Not easy! Nevertheless they manage!'

There. This is all I remember of Lacan's lecture: love amongst the hedgehogs.

Jean Delay, who had authorized Lacan to use his lecture room at Sainte-Anne, felt trapped in this venture. Each week, in his study, on the day of the seminar, he looked intently through his window at the parade, getting longer every time, of faithful pilgrims—the procession of followers. He was surprised at their number.

'It's not possible—after all, it isn't a tightrope walker!'

But nobody dared to say anything to the guru who drew so many people. However, one day we learnt that Lacan had chosen to leave Sainte-Anne to go to preach in the rue d'Ulm, at the senior college for the training of teachers. This departure was made with no noise, lost in the excitement to which the successes of the new chemotherapies for mental illness gave rise.

Presentation of the neuroleptics

To present these new therapeutics, Jean Delay had resolutely decided to integrate them into biology and to compare them with shock and aggressive methods.

Other times, other customs; five years beforehand it was the festival of the shock, the apotheosis of aggressive therapeutics. Now, what had been worshipped was being burned. On the basis of work that would be unearthed in the reports of the scientific societies, names now a little outdated were brandished: Reilly and Leriche, highlighting more recent research, in particular that of Laborit, slightly forgetting Huguenard. No longer was an aggressive approach to be used in the war against mental illness: the baton, stinging hydrotherapy, shocks, all had to be demobilized; neuroleptics and chlorpromazine brought relaxation, and with it, peace. Admittedly nothing had yet been found for melancholy, depression and anguish, but agitation, manic attacks, and some forms of delirium were cured, and hallucinations were disappearing.

All psychiatrists insisted upon the major qualities of the drugs; they worked without causing sleep, without damaging the mind, and without altering consciousness. Admittedly a certain indifference, a lack of interest, arose, but this affected the disagreeable elements in the patient's thoughts more than the requirements for normal behaviour. Reserpine, a little less active, also had similar qualities.

In his closely followed presentation, which had been greatly applauded at the Colloquium of 1955, Delay noted that shock therapies still had a role, in particular Sakel treatment in certain forms of schizophrenia, and electroconvulsive therapy in severe melancholias; but in his conclusion he outlined the perspectives of the future psychotropes:

'When penicillin was introduced in therapeutics,' he said, 'one saw afterwards much research developing which succeeded in the creation of many other antibiotics effective against very different germs. One can hope that it will be the same with the new psychotropes, and that after chlorpromazine and reserpine, other drugs will be found which will act in a specific manner in different mental illnesses.'

The new psychopharmacological research was set to prove him completely right.

Neuroleptics and psychopharmacology

The psychoses, mental illnesses, are the broken destinies of those who have followed paths they did not choose for themselves. Even if they thought of following their leanings, they have been pushed by urges veiled in mystery until delirium gradually developed. In adopting behaviour dictated by unusual impulses, they built up an edifice that has gradually become transformed into a citadel, where their lost reason is not regained and they are isolated beyond recall.

The walls of this fortress, so difficult to besiege with psychotherapy, and which the shock therapies had so much difficulty in weakening, had been breached and undermined by the neuroleptics, little by little reaching the person within.

The short-term and long-term effects of neuroleptics

The development of a psychosis in a mental patient follows several stages prior to final derangement, but these stages are not all passed through right away. Thus what especially struck the experimenters was the short-term action of the neuroleptics, which developed rapidly, and which was essentially sedative. On sleep, the neuroleptics act indirectly by paralysing the sleep control organ, which is in the brain, and is called the anterior reticular substance.

The most characteristic effect of these drugs is their capacity to reduce manic excitation and agitation; this distinguishes them from the 'minor tranquillizers' of which we will speak later, which are not capable of producing such results.

The neuroleptics intervene also in an 'incisive' manner in the acute psychoses. In fact, this was no longer a purely sedative action, working like a 'chemical straitjacket' (the term is absolutely wrong in this case), but on the contrary a process of restoration of lucidity, with progressive diminution in delirium and even hallucinatory activity, and an improvement in contact with the patients.

The use of neuroleptics in continuous treatment has made it possible for patients to leave their asylums, where otherwise they would have to spend the rest of their lives. Administration of these drugs has completely transformed the chronic psychoses.

The construction of a psychosis or a delirium does not happen in one day; it is not made from monolithic blocks of delirious ideas, but rather, like the tomb of Antiochus, from thousands, millions of aggregated micropsychoses, like the round pebbles of the King of Commagene's mausoleum. For the first time, neuroleptic drugs provide a way to fragment, break up, this construction; and the erosion of the patient's absurd convictions ends in a slow but profound reorganization of his or her mental make-up.

If you read the classic treatises written by the celebrated psychiatrists of former times—Jean Esquirol, Jean Falret, Gaston de Clérambault—you see that if the signs and symptoms of dementia described by these authors are still valid, the progress of the disease is completely changed. Thanks to the neuroleptics, the psychoses no longer follow the classic pattern of years ago.

Since the 1950s, the systematic use of neuroleptics has transformed the conditions and the therapy, and also the need for hospitalization in chronic delirium, making treatments possible that are now provided outside the 'concentration camp' atmosphere of the asylum. I have never understood the paradoxical attitude of some asylum psychiatrists who at the same time recognize the interest of these drugs and yet deny that they represent an advance. Henri Ey himself, in one of the last articles he wrote on the neuroleptics and the hospital psychiatric services, bears witness to an attitude that is irritatingly ambivalent.

After relating his version of the story of the neuroleptics, after praising their qualities, their efficacy, their surprising effects on the delirious and chronic psychoses, their extraordinary hallucinolytic power; after having acknowledged the fact that, in spite of its detractors, 'chemotherapy cannot be prohibited, that it must be prescribed for its antipsychotic power' as if suddenly he saw in this confession a risk of dishonest compromise, he begins his final summary with this sentence, which is, to say the least, surprising: 'It is not true that the introduction of the phenothiazines, and notably chlorpromazine in 1952, had revolutionized the psychiatric hospitals.' He goes on to explain that progress had begun in reality at the beginning of the century with the introduction of ergotherapy (patients given daily tasks to keep them occupied) and afterwards was confirmed with the shock treatments. But Henri Ey had to end by admitting that in his own department at Bonneval, between 1921 and 1937 he recorded 6% of discharges of schizophrenia and chronic delirium patients, compared with 67% between 1955 and 1967.

Throughout the world the statistics were unanimous. There was a veritable exodus of the intramural psychiatric population from the asylums. The population of the psychiatric hospitals, which had been growing by 7% per annum, only grew by 4.3% in 1955 and 2.5% in 1956. Between 1955 and 1968, the number of mental patients hospitalized in the USA dropped by 30%. In 1955 in France, 18% of admissions to psychiatric hospitals were office admissions (required by the administrative authorities or the police). In 1966, there were only 12% office admissions, and in 1976 the figure was 2%.

These results are not only due to the effects of the chemotherapy of mental illness, but also the result of improvements in concepts of supervision and information in the clinics, dispensaries and institutes of mental hygiene. However, the new drugs have contributed greatly to this progress, and this has to be recognized.

The attitude of people who were unconvinced by or opposed to these drugs is curious; perhaps they felt it wrong to endorse something they did not understand. Nevertheless, they could see how neuroleptic therapy had changed mental illness, the patients, the asylums and the psychiatrists.

The modification of mental illness by neuroleptics

Mental patients, often project their illness, exteriorize it, follow it and sometimes wish to share it with others. It is then that they disturb and strike out at society, which, wrongly or rightly, considers them a danger to themselves or others, and has them admitted.

Now, under the influence of psychotropic drugs and neuroleptics, these active deliriums become 'encysted'; we no longer see their explosion and the consequences they bring. Not only does the patient no longer follow the delirium or show abnormal behaviour, but instead of speaking frequently about these hallucinations, the patient becomes reticent and refuses to recall the delirious ideas. Little by little, under the influence of the drugs, these patients become uninterested in what had previously occupied all their thoughts and the whole field of their consciousness: as they become first tired of, then indifferent to the harassment of their delirium, these hallucinations gradually fade away, all the quicker since they will be less turned over, less pondered over: it is not unusual for patients to come to make fun of their strange thoughts, which although still as deeply felt, now appear insignificant. Removed from pathological preoccupations, the patient regains interest in other values, nearer to the reality of the rest of the world.

So a normalization of behaviour is seen, which makes it possible for the patient to reintegrate into society.

Cure or relapse

It is only when patients are able to criticize their former mental state and behave solely in an appropriate manner that one can speak of lasting improvement or even of cure. But beware! The need to continue the treatment is imperative. The chronic psychoses that used to fill the asylums are now calmed by the neuroleptics, but their roots are in many cases as resistant as those of couch grass. One of the most striking aspects of the neuroleptics—one that demonstrates their activity—is the return of delirium and the frequency of relapse and second offences when treatment is interrupted or the dosage is reduced.

The quality of the results obtained with neuroleptics is influenced by the reception the patient receives on discharge from hospital. A caring family environment, supervision by a cooperative doctor, assuring control of the regular taking of medication, are good prognostic factors, compared with the risk run by a patient living alone, with no supportive person to check the administration of the treatment.

This is why the introduction of prolonged-action neuroleptics represents an unquestionable advance in achieving true effectiveness with the smallest doses.

The moral problem of long-acting neuroleptics

It is undeniable that the act of administering an intramuscular injection of neuroleptic drug every three or four weeks to provide therapeutic continuity and effective cures has been a considerable step forward in the treatment of chronic psychoses. However, the ease with which this treatment can be imposed has concerned psychiatrists. Some wondered whether one had the right, even in the patient's interest, to treat by the strength of a single injection a recalcitrant, delirious patient or a schizophrenic patient oblivious to the illness.

In truth, this problem arises not only with long-acting neuroleptics but with all treatments imposed on a mentally ill and oblivious patient, whose opinion is difficult to ask. What makes the problem more acute, however, for these neuroleptic injections is that the doctor's responsibility must be exercised, carefully evaluating the risks and chances of success of long-term treatment. It is therefore for the doctor to judge, in the patient's interest, the effect or the therapeutic ineffectiveness. This is why psychiatrists must keep their freedom of prescription, to offer it or refuse it, in accordance with their conscience. As Henri Ey emphasized, 'the neuroleptic, and particularly the long-acting neuroleptic, should not be prescribed as an alibi, as a surreptitious way of leaving it to something else to take care of somebody.'

LSD and the neuroleptics

A cup of tea. Andrée G had insisted on swallowing the drug in a cup of tea, but not any old tea.

'I want Lapsang Souchong!'

She said this smiling and looking at Dr Hiroshi Nakajima, who was smiling back at her.

'What are you two plotting?'

'Hiroshi has to go to Birmingham to get ready for your visit to Elkes and Mayer-Gross; if you let me go with him we will go through London. I know where you can find Lapsang Souchong. I'll bring a packet back and I'll be the guinea pig.'

This time I understood; my two collaborators were keen to spend a weekend together in London.

'I can buy a packet if you give me the address.'

The discretion and the very Japanese politeness of Hiroshi Nakajima made him propose this solution, which he obviously did not wish for.

I gave the requested leave and now we have at the laboratory some fine packets of tea, the green packets of Fortnum and Mason, Piccadilly. As for me, I have my packet of Earl Grey, perfumed with bergamot, and Andrée G gets me to taste her Lapsang Souchong—'the tea with the famous smoky flavour'. I confess that I do not appreciate this terribly smoked China tea very much.

'You'll see, it is very good, without sugar. We'll drink some tomorrow. If you like, I'll be ready for the experiment.'

Several weeks ago, I had already checked everything: the effective doses have been worked out, the mixture of the products has been studied *in vitro*, that is to say in an apparatus, and *in vivo*, on animals. There is, and will be, no risk. Obviously, there is always the same anguishing worry when making the leap from the test tube or from the mouse or rat to a human being. Nevertheless, I want to know, and I want to confirm what I have observed on pieces of living tissue, on organs kept alive, on the behaviour of laboratory animals, and on my turning mice. I have seen that all the signs and all the reactions provoked by LSD on biological tests or on pharmacological trials are abolished, counteracted or inhibited by chlorpromazine, which calms agitated patients and reduces psychoses.

On animals whose reactions had been rendered abnormal by the processes about which I have spoken previously, chlorpromazine worked marvellously; the animals became calm again, and their behaviour normal. What I wanted to see now was the action of chlorpromazine on an experimental human psychosis provoked by LSD.

According to my experiments in the laboratory, chlorpromazine should counteract the action of LSD or make it disappear. This is what I am going to check on Andrée G, my collaborator who, already a volunteer for a previous experiment with LSD, is willing to do it again, this time receiving chlorpromazine as well, to study the antagonist action of the neuroleptic on psychological disorders provoked by LSD. We have all the data from the preceding test and we can thus compare the two trials.

It is Andrée G who wanted to make the tea. We provided a one-litre glass laboratory beaker, where she infused her smoked tea; but to repeat the experiment in the same conditions as the previous time, she swallowed 150 micrograms of LSD with pure water. About forty minutes after taking this, she warned us, 'Children, here it is. I'm taking off.'

We waited a little, then gave her an intramuscular injection of chlorpromazine. The result was astonishing. Although the psychological disorder provoked by the first time by LSD had lasted more than eight hours, no more than twenty minutes had elapsed after the chlorpromazine injection before Andrée G had become almost normal again. Admittedly, the mixture in her body of LSD and chlorpromazine did not leave her with a perfect physical receptiveness; a few feelings of unsteadiness, a heavy sensation in the limbs, a thirst which she quenched by drinking her smoky tea—all this bore witness to the toxic action of the LSD–chlorpromazine cocktail. In contrast, on the mental plane there was no disassociation, no loss of thought control, no disorientation nor distortion of time or place. Chlorpromazine, by its neuroleptic action, had practically swept away all the hallucinogenic power of the LSD, confirming my experimental findings that this drug was a powerful antagonist of LSD.

Denber subsequently confirmed that chlorpromazine was also an antagonist of the hallucination provoked by mescaline, the peyote alkaloid.

Certainly it was already known that chlorpromazine lessened and often abolished the hallucinations of mental patients, but this was a fine demonstration a posteriori of its powerful activity on psychoses provoked by chemical poisons. This observation did not greatly clarify the mechanism by which chlorpromazine could work, but permitted the problem of the production of psychoses to be approached with some interesting hypotheses.

The mysteries of mental illness

The absence of consensus about mental illness, its merits or its dangers, its legitimacy or its prohibition in our society, its acceptance as an illness by psychiatry, or its rejection by anti-psychiatry, does not diminish the problem of its existence, of its forms, and above all of its appearance. The 'appearance' of mental illness, in the sense that it arises unexpectedly, adding itself to a customary thought, which it disrupts and alters, raises the question of its origin, and the triggering cause of this psychological modification.

It is natural to think that even if an unforeseen event has set off mental illness, two elements are equally involved: a more or less susceptible mind, and more or less disturbing disruptions or changes. It is possible, with examinations, psychological analyses and mental tests, to measure the qualities and performance of a mind, but the most powerful microscopes and the most extensive laboratory analyses have never been able to detect any indication of mental illness in the cells of the brain or in biochemical reactions.

Which microbes and viruses cause infectious diseases, and which excessive or reduced chemical reactions block the arteries, jam the joints, weaken the bones, or cause calculus formation in the kidneys or gallbladder, are well known. The factor that triggers cancer is unknown, but we know how to detect and recognize cancer cells, tumours can be seen to develop and enlarge, and cancerous tissue can even be cultivated. In contrast, nobody knows what triggers off mental illness, and when it is present, as evidenced by delirium, hallucination, shouts, and cries of rage, nothing abnormal can be found in the blood or organs of the patient. If by chance the patient dies in an accident or from some other illness, the autopsy reveals the lesions produced by the accident or illness; but no cell in the whole body, including all the parts of the brain, will reveal why the patient became mentally ill.

However, between the years 1948 and 1953, two fundamental facts were discovered in psychiatric medicine:

- With well-defined chemical products like LSD 25 and mescaline (peyote alkaloid) hallucinations, delirium, and psychological disorders resembling mental illness can be provoked in humans.
- With medication prepared with the aid of well-defined chemical products (chlorpromazine, reserpine), some hallucinations and delirium can be arrested, and some mental illnesses can be cured. It is also possible, with these same products, to abolish the experimentally induced psychoses and mental illnesses provoked by LSD 25 and mescaline.

There was an obvious conclusion: mental illness developing spontaneously in some patients could be caused by chemical or biological disturbances which are as yet undetectable, either on their own or through the damage they have done, which likewise passes unnoticed.

Biochemical concepts of psychoses and psychopharmacology

It matters little how the soul is viewed, but organs and their function have to be used to feel, want and think, and as the function determines the organ, it follows that if not the soul then at least the thought must be located in the brain. What is more, why look anywhere else? It is therefore at the level of the brain that the actions of poisons like LSD and drugs like chlorpromazine have been studied.

The anatomy of the different parts of the brain studied under the microscope, as I have already said, has revealed nothing. The chemical constituents of the brain were also examined, their respective proportions measured out, and there again everything was normal. No difference could be detected between a normal individual and a hallucinated delirious patient, between the brain of a sane individual and a brain intoxicated with LSD or permeated with chlorpromazine.

So, one returns to the study of the primitive mechanisms of neurology, the first studies carried out to explain nerve impulse transmission—in other words, the physiology of the nervous system and the physical and particularly the chemical conditions of its function.

In order not to get lost on this astonishing investigative journey, I am going to use simple images—simplistic, the experts will say—to explain neurochemistry.

From neurochemistry to neuropsychopharmacology

It is known that the nerve impulse is analogous to an electric current, and it is also known that the nerve and brain demonstrate this electric current, which can be picked up, measured and recorded with apparatus such as the electroencephalograph. This nerve impulse is propagated in the brain and in the nerve cells and their extensions by the intermediary of chemical substances that are continually being formed and broken down, destroyed and modified, then renewed like the elements and chemical products in a battery or an accumulator. The brain and nerves manufacture these substances, which were called first neurohormones, then nerve impulse mediators, then neurotransmitters, and finally monoamines.

They all have names, some generally known, some less so: histamine, acetylcholine, serotonin, tryptamine, dopamine, noradrenaline and adrenaline. These products were first detected in the body, then they were localized to different parts of the brain and the nerves. Next they were isolated, then synthesized, and thus available in larger quantities, they were administered to animals and humans. Their sites of action and their responses to hallucinogenic chemical substances like LSD and drugs like chlorpromazine were also studied.

The result of all this research? In the end, something was found, thanks to these neurochemical studies. It has been possible to analyse the mechanism of action of the monoamines at the level of the cells that give rise to them, and at the level of the receptors that capture them, retain them or release them. Although the way in which delirium and schizophrenia develop is not yet understood, the way neuroleptics act on these monoamines and inhibit or reinforce their action has been seen.

Thanks to these studies in neurochemistry it has been possible partly to explain the mechanism of action of hallucinogenic products (LSD, mescaline) and to focus on experimental psychiatry methods based on cerebral biochemistry. The features that a chemical molecule must comprise to be active in psychiatry have also been characterized *a posteriori*. Thus modifications of animal behaviour and modifications of the cerebral metabolism of the neurotransmitters under the influence of neuroleptics have enabled the introduction of a new pharmacology appropriate for the development and study of chemical substances likely to become active medications in therapeutic psychiatry. This is what, in 1956, in a study published in the *Semaine des Hôpitaux de Paris*, and that summarized my work, I called, with Jean Delay, *psychopharmacology*.

The first steps in psychopharmacology

The word 'psychopharmacology', the American Ann E. Caldwell tells us, has been in use for a long time. Anglo-Saxon authors—March in 1920 and Thornes in 1935—had used the term in scientific communications. It is also certain that without knowing it, and without specifying it by this term, when Paracelsus prescribed laudanum, Pinel opium, Moreau de Tours hashish, Paul Guiraud promethazine and Deniker chlorpromazine for mentally ill patients, they were all employing psychopharmacology: they were studying and making use of the action of these drugs on the human mind. In this sense, the term means no more than the expression 'medicinal therapy in psychiatry'.

What I hoped to indicate in 1956, by introducing the term 'psychopharmacology' in France, was that a new chapter in pharmacology dedicated to psychotropic drugs was opening. I considered that the discovery of 'mind poisons' like hallucinogens (LSD, psilocybin, STP) and 'mind medications' like the neuroleptics (chlorpromazine, reserpine) filled a void, that of *psychiatric pharmacology*, and that research, manufacture, use and study of the mechanisms of action of these psychotropic drugs would be the realm of *psychopharmacology*.

By now, collaboration between the clinical psychiatrists who studied mental illness at the patient's bedside and those who like me researched the fundamental problems posed by the psychoses in the laboratory had become so close that we exchanged our ideas and white coats irrespective of discipline. Every new drug put forward by the drug companies was studied on our experimental animals, and from our laboratory results also came forth from which new therapeutic molecules were derived.

Deniker has called this period 'the golden age of psychopharmacology', and I am certainly not going to contradict him.

The term 'psychopharmacology' did not always meet with immediate approval. I remember Professor Delay telling me about a criticism from the pharmacologist Hazard at the Academy of Medicine, who had asked him what psychopharmacology was. In fact, for a few years, *traditional pharmacologists understood nothing about psychopharmacology*. As for the traditional psychiatrists, they only adopted it with time, and after reading the advertising leaflets from the pharmaceutical product laboratories.

Nevertheless, the special techniques focused upon in my laboratory and the therapeutic results obtained by Deniker attracted foreign doctors and scientists to study this new science of psychopharmacology.

And so, at Sainte-Anne, in Jean Delay's department, a large number of students and researchers from all over the world were recruited. The Japanese were particularly numerous, and after the departure of the pharmacologists and psychiatrists Kumaga, Kobayashi and Akimoto, I had the pleasure of having as a pupil the young Kurihara, later a professor of psychiatry in Japan, and particularly Hiroshi Nakajima, who was my assistant for ten years, married one of my French collaborators, and having been chief of the drugs department of the World Health Organization at Geneva, became director of that body for the whole Asian region.

It was with Hiroshi Nakajima that we were the first to show the fundamental differences existing between the principal drugs acting on the nervous system. A sedative, a hypnotic, a tranquillizer and a neuroleptic each have different actions in animals, which can now be distinguished thanks to tests we refined during that period. Each of these products produces different behaviour patterns, which make it possible to classify them before their use in humans.

We were among the first to demonstrate the action of the neuroleptics and psychotropes on monoamines and neurotransmitters. Thanks to these theoretical studies I could schedule work with chemists, asking them for molecules, which they succeeded in synthesizing and which I then studied in animals before trying them in humans. In this way a collaboration developed between my psychopharmacology laboratory and Dr Paul Rumpf's Centre of Applied Organic Chemistry at the National Centre of Scientific Research (CNRS). A psychochemistry department was established there, directed by the chemist with green eyes who had prepared the Antabuse for my thesis, and who in the meantime had become my wife.

This work was officially recognized by the establishment in 1960 of the first institute in the world carrying the name of psychopharmacology: the

Neuropsychopharmacology Research Unit of the National Institute of Health and Medical Research (Institut National de la Santé et de la Recherche Médicale—INSERM), of which I was made scientific director. Official funds were obtained for the construction of this institute. The building, originally conceived within Sainte-Anne, encroached on the road, and it was decided to knock down the wall, which no longer served any purpose there. When the enclosing wall of Sainte-Anne was demolished at the junction of the rue d'Alésia and the rue de la Santé, Mendelsohn, the architect directing the works, remarked jokingly to me that if Pinel had set free the in-patients at the Salpêtrière, it had taken psychopharmacology to bring down the wall of Sainte-Anne. It was in fact the first breach made in the high enclosing wall since its construction.

From this collaboration between my institute at Sainte-Anne, the psychiatric department of Delay and Deniker, and that of chemistry which my wife directed, a series of therapeutic achievements was to flow.

Official recognition of psychopharmacology

When Ann Caldwell, the librarian from Bethesda in the USA, tells us that the word 'psychopharmacology' has been known for a long time, I wish she could have been present at the scientific gatherings that took place on this theme between the years 1953 and 1957. Until 1956, she would only have heard this term spoken by my collaborators and myself, but she would also have been able to see that it was as badly received by the clinical psychiatrists as by the pharmacologists. The former declared that I had forgotten psychiatry, and the latter, that I had no right to tag pharmacology on to psychiatry.

At the colloquium on neuroleptics organized at Sainte-Anne in October 1955, Delay and Deniker, who presided at the gathering, never pronounced this word. As for me, I contented myself with organizing a series of demonstrations in my laboratory using my turning mice, fighting Siamese fish and the behavioural reactions of various animals. I had labelled this demonstration 'Experimental Psychopharmacology'.

The pharmacologist Reuse, from Brussels, who was present at the colloquium, had been interested in my experiments and was one of my first supporters. I was especially happy over the long, attentive visit that Professor Mayer-Gross paid me, at the end of which he invited me to lecture at the experimental psychiatry centre that he directed with Joel Elkes in Birmingham.

'You must tell us about your psychopharmacology,' he told me.

The experimental psychiatry centre at Birmingham

I only knew Willy Mayer-Gross, who was one of the great figures in psychiatry in the first half of the century, a very little. He was already well known and appreciated in Germany, where he had been professor of psychiatry and joint director of the clinic at Heidelberg, and where he had founded, with Beringer, the famous journal *Nervenartz*. Driven out by the Nazis, he had found refuge in London in 1933 where he successively worked at the Maudsley Hospital, then at the Crichton, and at the end of his career in Birmingham, where he had established an experimental psychiatry centre with Joel Elkes.

What fascinated me about this centre was that all the disciplines were united there to work towards a better understanding of mental illness.

The extraordinary psychiatric knowledge of Mayer-Gross, who had been a pioneer in all the therapies (insulin, cardiazol and electroconvulsive) as well as in experimental psychosis techniques (LSD, mescaline) was associated with that of the most eminent collaborators: Ginzel in biochemistry, Bradley in electroencephalography, and especially Joel Elkes, who coordinated all these fields of learning oriented towards psychiatry.

When Mayer-Gross introduced me before my lecture, he told the listeners from the University of Birmingham who were present:

'From everything that will be said to you this evening, bear in mind this new word: psychopharmacology. We already practise it here without realizing it, and everything we do tomorrow and in the future, everything we will want to do, will be gathered into this new discipline about which you are now going to hear.'

Mayer-Gross, despite his advanced age, still had an extraordinary facility for adaptation to every new idea, and he held very sound views on the future of psychiatry. So, using new treatments with neuroleptics, he founded a day hospital at Uffculme, near Birmingham, which was a model of its kind.

The Germans in 1960 restored both his property and his post at the University of Heidelberg, with its honorarium, as well as awarding him the directorship of a research institute. He told us that he had asked that this institute should be called a psychopharmacology laboratory. He was getting ready to return to Germany when death cruelly overtook him on 15 February 1961.

The open-mindedness which Mayer-Gross had shown towards psychopharmacology was not repeated everywhere, and many scientific meetings would only accept this new discipline in their programmes with reluctance. Nevertheless, I managed to introduce it in the international neurochemistry symposia.

A symposium at Aarhus

When Joel Elkes had invited me to take part in the first neurochemistry symposium at Aarhus, I had to consult an atlas to find out where this town was—which I have never forgotten since 1956.

Before the congress, my wife and I had made a tour of Scandinavia, and visited Arvid Carlsson's laboratory at the University of Gothenburg.

He was beginning his work on the metabolism of the amino acids. Passing through Norway, north of Oslo, on the edge of Lake Mjøsa, I had wanted to see the catlin fishermen who blew their reed pipes while hauling in their nets.

During the whole journey we hardly ever ate anything other than potatoes and fish (mostly herring) in sweet sauces. At Aarhus, attending the cocktail party for the symposium opening, we found yet again, on pretty canapés, a thousand varieties of herring marinades, mostly sweetened with sugar. I was hesitating over choosing another sample of the fish when a kind, blond young man offered to help me pick out some unsweetened herring. This was the assistant to Professor Erik Strömgren, our host at the Aarhus University Institute of Psychiatry.

At one point the person I was speaking to, who appeared to have a great knowledge of French psychiatry, told me about the descent of Gaeten de Clérambault, who, by marriage with the Marsay family, was descended in a straight line from René Descartes' mother. I knew, of course, of the work of Clérambault, chief physician at the Special Infirmary of the Prefecture of Police in Paris, but I knew nothing of his relationship to Descartes. Strömgren's assistant seemed greatly interested in Clérambault.

'I do not understand,' he told me, 'how this great French psychiatrist came to do his doctoral thesis on an otorhinology subject.'

This question, which perhaps would have left other doctors dumb, quickly triggered my reply.

I knew the answer. First of all, it was not an otorhinology thesis; it was a psychiatry thesis on 'the otohaematoma of mentally ill patients'. At one time I had been interested in the 'nonsensical symptoms' of mental patients; disorders which for decades had been put down to mental illness but which in reality were only problems resulting from the patient's life circumstances. Clérambault's thesis on this subject was a remarkable critical observation on a deformity of the ear, often seen in mental inpatients, up till the end of the nineteenth century. Everybody knew about the cauliflower ear of boxers, fighters and wrestlers. This deformity arises from blows to the ears, which cause haemorrhages (otohaematomas); secondarily, these change the shape of the cartilage of the ear. Now, it was thought that the cauliflower ears of mental patients were a sign of their mental illness, whereas Clérambault showed that they were deformed by repeated blows which mental patients had formerly suffered, or which they gave themselves in striking their heads against the walls of their cells.

This explanation given to Strömgren's assistant did not prevent me from remarking that the herring he had picked out for me was just as sugared as the rest, and I informed him of my vexation. He apologized, and reassured me, 'This evening, at the banquet, there is chicken with gratin potatoes. It was me who chose the menu.'

All the first part of the gala meal was sweetened, including the mayonnaises which went with the fish. When the chicken arrived, the head waiter served me with a drumstick, and some nice potatoes which were not gratin but looked fine. They had been well fried, but powdered sugar had been added to the hot butter.

When I told my new friend of my disappointment with the sweet chicken, we burst into laughter, and when I told him that in spite of all these Scandinavian sweets I was not going to sink into a depression, he suddenly said, 'You know, now, with Largactil, we calm down and treat manic agitation perfectly, but I believe there is a remarkable cure for depression. I have been trying it successfully for several months. It is an old remedy used by an Australian and which French psychiatrists also tried, and now everybody has forgotten about it. But I myself find that it is extraordinary.'

The young Aarhus psychiatrist also added, a little disappointedly, 'My chief doesn't believe in it much. Others will have to try it.'

When I asked him what he was referring to, he told me almost apologetically, 'Oh, just lithium carbonate.'

Returning to Paris a week later, I confess I was still thinking of the sweetened herrings but I had quite forgotten about the lithium carbonate of the young Danish psychiatrist, whose name was Mogens Schou; it was to take more than ten years to demonstrate the remarkable activity of lithium and so to offer psychiatric therapeutics one of the best mood-regulating drugs.

At neurochemical gatherings, there was little talk about the clinic, illnesses and pharmacology. Everything reported came out of studies done in test tubes, analysers, centrifuges and sophisticated biochemical apparatus. The results were expressed as oxygen consumption, cellular respiration, energy measurement after incubation, and ultracentrifugation. Interest was taken in the metabolism of the nerve cell and its maintenance within the nerve and in the brain; and this cerebral substance, this greasy, whitish mass—we have about a kilo of it in our cranial cavity— was little by little explored, probed and analysed, looking within it for a few mines, a few seams, for research.

I often spent exultant days with these neurochemical pioneers, tossing ideas about, and manipulating hypotheses into which we threw the basis of what was to become neuropharmacology.

As for me, I reasoned 'broadly', as my colleagues said, and they 'in detail'. These discussions were compered by Heinrich Waelsch, a specialist in amino acids, Seymour S. Kety, who with Francis Schmidt was one of the first to have measured cerebral metabolism, and the British researchers Derek Richter and Herman Blaschko. Often reserved, but full of fun in these shows, the American Julius Axelrod sometimes gave us imitations of Stanley Laurel. One day he said to me, 'I am going to come and work with you for a sabbatical year.'

And when I laughingly asked him what good he would be able to do in my laboratory, he answered, 'I am good at making a dry martini.'

He also knew how to manipulate the cerebral monoamines with which he succeeded in explaining a large part of the mechanism of nerve impulse transmission, which a few years later earned him the Nobel prize for medicine.

The year of psychopharmacology: 1957

In the success of a discovery, only twenty-five per cent is due to the invention itself: the rest is development. This may seem surprising, but it is true. It is because this principle is not appreciated that many inventions are left in desk drawers.

The discovery of the hallucinogens (LSD), the neuroleptics (chlorpromazine) and the relationship between cerebral neurochemistry and behaviour modified by psychological drugs had since 1950–2 brought about a climate, an ambience, in which clinicians and laboratory researchers were keen to collaborate.

All of this had to be brought together, and integrated: results had to be presented, interest for this research had to be stimulated by showing its pragmatic value, a demand had to be developed and a market created. This job of marketing was wonderfully understood by the pharmaceutical companies.

Psychopharmacology and marketing

Apart from a few aspirin tablets, antibiotics, and possibly some cough linctus, the pharmacy of a psychiatric asylum mainly had a stock of phenobarbitone and hypnotics, anti-epileptics, and sedatives of all kinds; but correctly speaking, no specifically psychiatric drugs. It was the same the world over. Mentally ill patients represented a category whose illness had no remedy, except the routine medicines for times when they suffered from a physical affliction like anybody else might do.

Now, the results obtained with chlorpromazine and reserpine showed by their specificity that millions of mental in-patients, and many others as well, could now be regularly dosed with drugs that had been specially prepared for them. A new market was opening up to the pharmaceutical industry, and it dived in. Already Spécia in France, with Largactil, was solicited by laboratories throughout the world wanting licensing contracts, and Ciba in Switzerland, which was assured of the monopoly of the manufacture of reserpine, tightly regulated its sale.

The great industrial groups of pharmaceutical laboratories at once saw the commercial interest of the discovery of new psychotropic drugs, and directly or indirectly set up research in this direction. It is certain that these investments were for motives of profit, but it would be wrong to reproach these industries, which achieved ninety per cent of the new discoveries in drug materials.

And so, beginning in the year 1955, numerous contacts were made between researchers in the industry and the university hospital centres throughout the world. Scientific meetings, publications, and research were subsidized by the laboratories which through information channels and the mass media spread the news that mental illness could be effectively treated. Already official authorities were honouring and encouraging those who distinguished themselves in these paths of research.

The 1957 Lasker prizes

Each year the Albert Lasker Foundation in the USA rewards those who have made discoveries useful for humanity. These Lasker prizes recognize scientists who are often in the 'Nobelizable' category, thus backing up the idea that the Lasker prize is the American Nobel or pre-Nobel.

In 1957, the jury of the American Public Health Association awarded the Albert Lasker Reward, otherwise called the Lasker prize for medicine, to Pierre Deniker, Henri Laborit, Heinz Lehmann and Nathan Kline: the first three for their work on chlorpromazine, the fourth for his discovery of the antipsychotic action of reserpine.

This prize calls for a few comments from my point of view. First, the two Frenchmen Laborit and Deniker were rewarded in the United States, and that I know that no French authority, in 1957 or (I believe) for a long time afterwards, bothered to recognize their important discovery. Was Lehmann rewarded because he was the first in North America to report Deniker's experiments? I do not know. For Nathan Kline, his work on reserpine, certainly less effective than chlorpromazine, had introduced a drug into psychiatry that showed itself to be a remarkable psychopharmacological instrument.

If one examines the Nobel prizes for medicine awarded during the two decades prior to this Lasker prize, it is noticeable that they above all rewarded chemists and biochemists, the medical interest of whose research is still to be shown, or stands out poorly. This is why I think that the notice inscribed on the pedestal of the little statuette awarded to Deniker deserves to be better known:

'Accolade awarded for his introduction of chlorpromazine into psychiatry and his demonstration that a drug can influence the clinical evolution of the principal psychoses.'

The awarding in 1957 of the Lasker prize for medicine, firmly oriented towards the discovery of psychotropic drugs, would give rise to other scientific demonstrations in this same direction. The most specific and most important was to be the international symposium on psychotropic drugs organized under the direction of Professor Emilio Trabucchi in Milan.

Trabucchi's symposium

Emilio Trabucchi was an out-of-the-ordinary character who has shaped a whole generation of the best Italian doctors, biologists, and pharmacologists.

I had met him in Milan, in his huge pharmacology institute. He received his visitors in an extraordinary study, which scientists from all over the world still remember. It was an immense room largely occupied by a disproportionately enormous desk, buried under books, records and reports, which was extended with tables where there were piled up more stacks of reviews, journals and encyclopaedias. To break up these alignments and this chaos of paperwork, from the middle of all these documents, stalks, branches, leaves and flowers of a great variety of ornamental plants sprang from cleverly positioned vases. In this tangle of scientific literature and greenhouse vegetation, Emilio Trabucchi knew exactly where to retrieve the document, article or letter he needed for his work or for conversation with his visitor.

Conversation with him was not only pleasant, but friendly and warm. Very soon we were guided from the jungle of his desk towards a clearing arranged in the room where we sat around a table to sample an excellent espresso. Depending on the subject being addressed, he called to collaborators in his institute who were working on the question to come and join in the discussion. His comments were always clear and precise, but he always let his pupils, whom he brought forward and to whom he entrusted responsibilities, have their say.

Researchers worldwide came to work in his laboratory, outstandingly well installed and equipped thanks to subsidies from the Italian state that his political connections, and also the national and international reputation of his institute, earned for him.

Emilio Trabucchi lived for his laboratory, for research, and for his students. A bachelor, he lived in a tiny room in his immense institute, a retreat where a monk would have felt cramped, and which harboured a few personal items, and, it was said, the one and only grey suit that he nearly always wore.

When Emilio Trabucchi had spoken to me about his project of organizing a congress on psychotropic drugs, he had particularly specified that his intention was to establish a close contact between clinical psychiatrists and the laboratory pharmacologists on this occasion.

'The psychiatrists, with the new psychosis medication, are all surprised by the powerful activity of these drugs. They do not know how they have come into their hands. Many are unaware that their discovery was due to the flair of clever clinicians and to fortuitous and unscientifically programmed circumstances. These clinicians, who get lost in the psychological analysis of the unexpected results they obtain, need to let us benefit from this experience so that we pharmacologists, in dialogue with them, can draw the necessary information from them so that we can find other drugs for them, this time specially designed for psychiatry. You have been,' he added, 'at the crossroads where psychiatry and pharmacology meet because of your training as a psychiatrist and your apprenticeship in pharmacology. Your example should be multiplied; it is in this spirit that new drugs for mental illness will be found.'

I talked to him about this psychopharmacology, which for me ideally achieved the collaboration that he hoped for.

'It has got to happen,' he told me, 'but the new word must be adopted officially by psychiatrists and pharmacologists by mutual consent. This is what I will try hard to achieve at my symposium, and you are going to help me.'

This is why the first world congress on psychopharmacology was located in Milan, but, the term not yet being in general use, it was officially entitled the International Symposium on Psychotropic Drugs.

This congress was outstandingly organized by two direct collaborators of Trabucchi, his pupils Silvio Garattini and Vittorio Ghetti.

Garattini put the programme together splendidly. He understood how to bring together the laboratory researchers most competent in the biochemistry, physiology and pharmacology of the brain and nerves, and also managed to select psychiatrists who knew how to talk about medicine—I would like to say the psychiatrists who did not use the verbiage and phraseology of the old asylum doctors.

Trabucchi's symposium on psychotropic drugs started on 9 May 1957, in the Via San Vittore in Milan. They used the symbol of the mandrake for the meeting—it appears on the frontispiece of the book that came out of the symposium.*

Our team from Sainte-Anne was represented by Deniker for the clinic, and my assistant Nakajima and myself for psychopharmacology. The Charenton hospital had sent Henri Baruk and his assistant Launay. Apart from Courvoisier and her collaborators Ducrot and Julou, who presented pharmacological studies for the Spécia laboratory, no French representative chaired any part of the meeting. They were not boycotting the symposium, but they had not yet grasped the importance of the new psychotropes, which, outside Sainte-Anne, only interested a few inquiring researchers like Jean Cahn and Monique Hérold. On the other hand, international participation was remarkable. Blaschko from Oxford explained the metabolism of the brain tissue mediators. Hoffer, the Canadian from Saskatoon, set out his celebrated theory of the origin of psychoses as a result of deviation of adrenaline metabolism. Denber, from New York, gave an analysis of all his experience with mescaline and LSD experimental psychoses, and their suppression by chlorpromazine administration. The Americans Claus Unna (from Chicago), Frank Ayd and Erminio Costa spoke about their clinical, pharmacological and electrophysiological experiments with the new drugs, and James Olds, from Los

---

* The proceedings were published as: Garattini S, Ghetti V, eds (1957) *Psychotropic Drugs.* Amsterdam: Elsevier.

Angeles, inventor of self-stimulation with implanted electrodes, showed that the neuroleptics suppressed this in all cases.

Other speakers were Park Shore and Bernard Brodie from Bethesda, forerunners of all the work on cerebral monoamines; Tripod and Alfred Pletscher from Basle; the future research director at Hoffmann-La Roche, Dieter Bente from Erlangen, William Feldberg from London; Vittorio Erspamer from Pisa (the Italian discoverer of serotonin); and Rothlin from Basle, the pharmacologist of LSD and the ergot alkaloids. Daniel Bovet, who had just been awarded the 1957 Nobel prize for medicine for his studies on the antihistamines and the curares, was also present with his assistant Vittorio Longo, to speak about the action of neuroleptics on the reticular substance.

This list of names may seem long and boring to many, but I am anxious to give it, for most of these experts were the true pioneers of psychopharmacology. Now partly forgotten, they are replaced in memory by other names of researchers who only repeated their experiments, while adding a few personal touches.

For, in fact, everything was said at this Milan symposium about the characteristics of the principal neuroleptic and tranquillizing psychotropes, with the exception of the antidepressants, which were still to be discovered. But with Pletscher, Shore and Brodie, the basis of the interpretation of the mechanism of action of all the psychotropes was established through their work on the monoamines.

Deniker presented an exhaustive study on results obtained with chlorpromazine. Baruk and Launay analysed their experiments with chlorpromazine in humans and monkeys. With Hiroshi Nakajima, I showed work bearing on the study of more than fifty psychotropic substances characterized by means of this special pharmacology that I am anxious to call 'psychopharmacology'. At the end of my presentation I showed a colour film to illustrate research showing that the psychotropes could be classified and differentiated, depending on their action on animals, as hypnotics, tranquillizers and antipsychotic neuroleptics, and that these same methods also made it possible to predict psychotonic and stimulant activity. Thanks to this forward-looking psychopharmacology, one could from then on test chemical molecules to identify their possible psychotropic properties and no longer have to rely on random tests as formerly.

From the Via San Vittore to La Scala

The Milan symposium took place in an extraordinary atmosphere. All the participants who met on this occasion already knew one another through their work, published in international reviews and distributed in all research centres. It was a time when there was something new to be found every month. Advances were being made over virgin territory with new ideas and new products: the administrative and legal restrictions of today did not exist. Instead of waiting several years before trying a new drug on humans, many experiments were carried out barely a few months after synthesis. Furthermore, the results obtained were so clear and decisive that the conclusions were only concerned with the formulation of constructive hypotheses, in place of the customary and tiresome contradictory discussions.

The warmth of the welcome by Trabucchi and his collaborators Garattini and Ghetti played a vital part in the success of this congress. The sessions were held in the completely new Leonardo da Vinci science and technology museum, in the former San Vittore convent. Before entering the conference room one went through vast corridors where all the prototypes of the great Leonardo were magnificently presented. In passing before these samples of ingenuity, which ranged from the most practical examples such as the weaving or weight-lifting machines and military devices, to utopian preconceptions of flying machines, we thought that, for us also, imagination was not lacking to safely find remedies for all forms of mental illness.

I have often gone back to Milan, and on many occasions have met Emilio Trabucchi, and his assistants Paoletti and especially Silvio Garattini, who now directs the Mario Negri Institute. The city is familiar to me, with its bustling centre near the Duomo, the Galleria Vittorio Emanuele and the Piazza Scala, and the quiet precincts of narrow streets leading towards the palaces, the parks with ornamental lakes where the old folks doze, and the ancient, deserted and sombre Romanesque churches. But the pleasure of these visits never surpassed that first occasion, better even than in de Sica's film *Miracle in Milan*, those remarkable three days that rewarded me a hundredfold for all my stubbornness and patience in holding on for the moment when there would be true drugs for mental illness. Drugs had now indeed been discovered: indeed, there were several of them. I had contributed to studying and refining them, and in Milan at last there was recognition by great scientists of the efforts made by all those who, like me, wanted the sick brain to have its medication, just like the heart, the liver and the kidneys. The search had to go on. It remained to find the remedy for anguish and mental pain to balance that for physical pain.

Apart from the Congress working sessions, breaks for relaxation had been planned to help us forget the preoccupations of our research. Emilio Trabucchi had organized an evening at La Scala for our benefit. For this gala he had reserved, long in advance, several rows of seats in the front, and if this had not been easy, it was even more difficult to get the Scala management to accept that the Congress participants would not be wearing the evening dress or dinner jacket usually called for in these places of honour. I remembered for a long time the scornful and haughty reception of the ushers, dressed as swordsmen and wrapped in chains, who showed us to our seats with a look of disgust.

We stayed at the Cavaliéri hotel on the Piazza Missori, near the Duomo, and thanks to Trabucchi we always had open table there. It was on 11 May 1957, during a lunch with Rothlin, Trabucchi, Deniker and Denber, that we had the idea of setting up a scientific society to extend this symposium, and to strengthen and multiply the relations and meetings between clinical psychiatrists and pharmacologists that had proved so effective in Milan.

Ernst Rothlin was in favour of this idea straight away. He was sure of the support of the four big Basle laboratories: Sandoz, of which he was scientific director, Hoffmann–La Roche, Ciba and Geigy. These laboratories, which represented between them ten per cent of the world's pharmaceutical production, were already engaged in psychotrope research and they all had observers in Milan.

We decided to form this new society on the occasion of the Second World Psychiatry Congress, which was to take place in Zürich at the beginning of September of the same year. We had three months to prepare the rules and the general constitutive assembly of a new group restricted to psychiatrists and pharmacologists, which we decided to call: the *Collegium Internationale Neuropsychopharmacologicum*—but for us, it was already the CINP.

The last survivor at the Second World Psychiatry Congress at Zürich

Why was Zürich chosen for the Second World Psychiatry Congress? Holding the Congress of 1950 in Paris was an obvious choice: we had good authors, mostly Parisian, fine patients, good doctors and good asylums; and rough-and-ready Paris, freed from the recent war, was enthusiastic, exuberant, tuned into topicality and innovation.

Seven years later, after the discovery of the neuroleptics, after chemical therapeutics turning upside down all the cure statistics, where should one go for a discussion? To Zürich! In this distinguished town, serious, of remote humour, mental illness was going to be talked about! Zürich, austere and thoughtful, but studious and wise, offered us in this month of September 1957, empty premises, because of the vacations of its celebrated Polytechnic.

It is sometimes best to avoid asking preposterous questions, so as to avoid the incongruity or oddity of the reply. I had asked Henri Ey why the Psychiatry Congress committee had settled on Zürich as the venue for the meeting. With a smile, he answered, 'Because they are not all dead!'

I smiled too, pretending to understand. I am still looking for the explanation, but I don't think it is worth it. In fact, all the Zürich psychiatrists I knew *had* died: Eugen Bleuler, the originator of the word 'schizophrenia'; Adolf Meyer, emigrated to the USA and father of American psychiatry, and Hermann Rorschach, the ink-blot test man. There remained one, however, whom I had forgotten, and who had survived all the others. He was very famous, known worldwide. But before speaking about him I would like to recount why the name of Hermann Rorschach reminds me of a misadventure.

The inventor of the ink-blot test, Hermann Rorschach, was born in Zürich in 1884. Few people know that his little schoolfriends already called him '*Kleck*', which means ink-blot. Some maintain that it was because his brother was an art teacher at his school, others because Hermann also drew with a pen. Contrary to these Zürich explanations, I think that the little Hermann owed his nickname to the scrawls with which he covered his fingers, lips and exercise books. His apprenticeship was beginning.

At the end of his schooling he studies medicine and ends up in Bleuler's department, in psychiatry at the Zürich Burghölzli. He has not forgotten his ink blots, he still makes them and shows them to his patients; he studies their reactions to these blots, which he squeezes between two sheets of paper, sometimes mixing inks of different colours. After making hundreds or thousands of blots, Rorschach chooses ten— five black and five coloured—and begins a massive operation involving displaying his blots and recording, transcribing, classifying and analysing the subjects' reactions to each of them.

For ten years Hermann 'the blot' applied his test to several hundred mental patients and a hundred normal people, and in 1921 he published his famous *Psychodiagnostic*, which is a treatise in which he explains his method and in which the ten blots are annexed, printed on cardboard. Eight months later, in 1922, Hermann Rorschach died; not from nervous exhaustion, but from appendicitis. This noted test of Rorschach's went around the world: it is famous, celebrated, and widely used. Perhaps because of the premature death of its author, further development was needed. A certain Bruno Klopfer set up the Rorschach International Institute to train 'Rorschach specialists' and distribute the book and cardboard plates printed with the famous blots.

Now I come to my misadventure.

In the 1950s, I went to learn how to use the Rorschach test from Madame Minkowska, an eminent psychology specialist who voluntarily lavished her teaching on the house physicians at Sainte-Anne. We were working with the only set of these plates, which were unobtainable at the time in France. There were ten of the celebrated blots printed on thick cardboard measuring eighteen centimetres by twenty-four centimetres. Wanting to study the reactions of a patient one day, I borrowed Minkowska's famous cards. Now the patient to whom I had shown them, taking advantage of a moment when I had been called to the telephone, destroyed three of them. He had folded them in two and immersed them in a pot of herbal tea. My annoyance was very great, and no less so were the difficulties I had to overcome to obtain, almost fraudulently, a model of the famous test published by Karger in Basle. I learnt that year that the

Swiss franc was a strong currency, and that the *Psychodiagnostic* and its ten plates were very expensive . . .

But enough about the ink-blot man; let us come back to the surviving and famous Zürich citizen, to this psychiatrist known throughout the world, about whom perhaps Henri Ey was thinking with his joke. This Zürich contemporary of Freud and of Bleuler, and who was still fully alive in 1957, was Carl Gustav Jung.

Jung knew everything, had learnt everything. He was reading Latin at the age of six, was acquainted with anthropology, Egyptology, the natural sciences and spiritualism; the latter before studying medicine. After a lecture given by Krafft-Ebing, he decided to specialize in psychiatry. Assistant to Eugen Bleuler, friend, then adversary, of Freud, it is Jung who, through his propaganda, gave psychoanalysis a worldwide dimension. Freud himself recognized this when he wrote to Karl Abraham: 'the arrival of Jung on the psychoanalysis scene has made the danger of seeing this science becoming a Jewish national affair remote.'

On bad terms with Freud until he died, Jung's polymath knowledge enabled him to mount an intelligent rebellion, and he trained some disciples. At the end of his life, he again became interested in the occult sciences: in 1944 he had written an essay, *Psychology and Alchemy*, in which he did not hesitate to tackle the enigmas of this science where chemistry and mystic speculations come together.

It was this extraordinary captivating personality whom I had the opportunity of meeting in Zürich.

Those who believe in it and those who don't

At the Second World Psychiatry Congress, the participants who had attended the earlier congress in Paris no longer recognized either the structure or the course they had followed seven years earlier. A break had been made, plain and clean, separating 'those who believe in it' from 'those who do not believe in it'—'it' being the new chemical therapies.

There were psychiatrists interested in the new therapies who had come to Zürich to learn more, and traditional psychiatrists, interested in the psychiatry of signs and symptoms, who continued to look upon the mentally ill patient as a plant to cultivate in the asylum greenhouse and to label in the herbarium of nosology. In the middle of these two persuasions—or rather from behind—the psychoanalysts circulated as if in a gymkhana.

In fact, the two poles of attraction at the Congress were the two symposia organized by Americans on the chemical origin of the psychoses and on the psychotropic drugs.

The first symposium was directed by Max Rinkel of Boston and H. C. B. Denber of New York. Rinkel and Denber had been amongst the first Americans to analyse experimental psychoses produced by mescaline and LSD. With Paul Hoch, they were also the first to study the antagonistic action of chlorpromazine on these chemical psychoses. The participants in the symposium were to talk of their experiments and develop their hypotheses on the production of psychoses by chemical substances. More than fifty communications had been listed in the programme on the chemistry of mind poisons, on the neurohumoral substances of the brain, on the blood of schizophrenic patients, and on oxidized adrenaline, which might be a brain toxin.

Scientists from Germany (who this time took part in the congress), Britain, Canada, Israel, the USA and Switzerland came to say that they had unsuccessfully sought the substance that, in the human body, could become altered so as to provoke mental illness. For France, Henri Baruk spoke of his long experience with catatonia and with bulbocapnine, and I myself presented work on new substances, synthesized by my wife from nicotinic acid, that reproduced psychoses. However, the great attraction of this symposium was the scientific personage chosen by Rinkel and Denber to direct the debates and discussion. This was an alert old man, with white hair and small spectacles; it was the great Zürich survivor, Carl Gustav Jung, who was then eighty-two years old. Although not attending the pure psychiatry sessions, and the display of work on psychoanalysis, he had agreed to preside over the least psychological and most organicist meeting of the Congress.

'I have come to your colloquium,' he said, 'because I know that my curiosity has some chance of being satisfied here: I shall learn some new things, and even if they turn out to be wrong later on, I will be able to dream or get off to sleep with them. And then you know, I believe in the possible origin of psychosis brought on by toxic substances. It is like the story of the fly without wings one sees walking. How could one believe that somebody had pulled them off. How could one believe that before this it could fly?'

The other symposium, organized by the American Nathan Kline, was to discuss the psychotropic drugs. There was a deployment of troops from all countries in the world who came to establish the efficacy of neuroleptics in mental illness; accounts were given of the results obtained using chlorpromazine and reserpine in all the psychoses. The throng was such that both the number of speakers and the length of their presentations had to be limited. Controversies were already arising over the descriptions and terminology of these products. Delay and Deniker could not get the term 'neuroleptic' adopted to describe the action of chlorpromazine. The weight and importance of the American delegates was strongly felt at the time. Although discovered in France, the action of chlorpromazine had become American property. Some foreigners believed (and still believe) in the American discovery of the neuroleptics. Hundreds, indeed thousands, of publications had appeared in the USA since 1953, and furthermore the Americans paid, in the form of grants, for work done abroad on subjects of research that they had taken on. Moreover, their considerable lead in biochemistry, neurochemistry and pharmacology had to be recognized. Assimilating the French discovery, they rapidly exploited it.

The research centres of the pharmaceutical laboratories also stood out in the discussions through the quality of their researchers.

At Kline's colloquium I presented an analysis of the properties of the psychotropic drugs based on their actions on the sympathetic, parasympathetic, central and peripheral nervous systems. This analysis, complemented with behavioural studies, enabled neuroleptic (on psychoses), tranquillizing (on certain neuroses), antidepressant and hypnotic actions to be distinguished. It is in everyday use today.

Between the rooms where the symposia of Kline and of Rinkel and Denber were going on, a small man who displayed exuberant vigour was seen in the Polytechnic corridors. This was Professor Ernst Rothlin. I remembered having met him several years previously at Sandoz, to show him my turning mice, then more recently at Trabucchi's symposium in Milan. A crack shot, and pistol champion in several Swiss cantons, he had invited me to see him in Basle, at 9 Sonnenweg, before the Congress, to show me his cups and trophies. He also had a remarkable collection of modern paintings, with magnificent canvases by Toulouse-Lautrec, Modigliani, Dufy and many other painters. At lunch, which we took together, he said to the maid who was awaiting the orders, 'We'll have the jar.'

It was a one-kilo jar of Beluga caviar, which we dug into with a ladle. He loved 'the little sturgeon's eggs' as he called them. He ate it unostentatiously.

Responsible for the pharmacological and clinical research of the Sandoz house, Rothlin was behind the great industrial development of the firm in the pharmaceutical sector. His work on the ergot alkaloids had made (and still makes) considerable profits for his employer. Like many researchers in the big Basle industries, he had been around the world many times, visiting his firm's subsidiary companies, research centres and universities. He spoke seven languages fluently, which provided him with a remarkable audience and enabled him to give lectures in many countries.

From the Polytechnic to the Zürich railway station buffet

In accordance with the decision and agreements made at Milan, Rothlin had prepared the Collegium's rules, and had circulated them to Denber, Deniker, Trabucchi and me.

Quite self-sufficiently, Rothlin had made up on his own a list of guests to be invited to the general assembly. In Zürich, he asked us for our suggestions for our respective countries, and between Kline's and

Rinkel and Denber's colloquia he had satisfactorily picked out worthy personalities.

We had decided to restrict membership of the Collegium to psychiatrists and pharmacologists well-versed in handling new brain drugs. In the case of psychiatrists the choice was easy. For the pharmacologists the selection was more difficult. The list was fiercely argued over. Emilio Trabucchi, who had come by train from Milan, had arrived with his own list, which was an impressive one. He wanted to have everybody in the Collegium, and maintained this was the only way to spread the new discipline.

Trabucchi spoke in French or Italian at our meetings, hardly knowing any other languages. When he was not happy about a proposition, he began by smiling, first saying everything was fine, but then explaining at length why he could not agree. In the end, everything was sorted out.

After our preliminary meeting, it was decided to hold the CINP constituent assembly in the Zürich railway station buffet. Ernst Rothlin had said one could get a good meal there, and that it was not expensive. Meantime, all the chosen members had received a personal invitation to this working meal. On 9 September at half-past eight the dinner took place, followed by a speech from Rothlin, tracing the history of our Milan initiative. He thanked Trabucchi, Deniker, Denber and me. He started his speech all over again in French, then in German, in Italian and in Spanish. At the end, one or two were yawning. The guests indicated by a show of hands their willingness to be founder members. Nobody withdrew. There was then a vote on adoption of the rules, then the nomination of an executive committee, of which I was one.

Some felt that the name 'Collegium Internationale Neuropsychopharmacologicum' was too long, and the Latin obsolete. However, all the founder members of the CINP present at the Zürich railway station buffet decided to assemble a first congress the following year. Emilio Trabucchi suggested it should be held in Italy, and stated that Rome would welcome us with open arms. The excellent facilities and perfect organization of his congress in Milan could only lead us to agree. To thank him for this, to show him our esteem, and to make taking official steps easier for him, he was unanimously elected President of the CINP. He had well deserved this.

As for me, I was happy. Of all the participating members, I, as both psychiatrist and pharmacologist, was able to appreciate better than anyone else the progress achieved. My adherence to clinical psychiatry and to pharmacological research had enabled me to see the achievement in ten years of what had first seemed almost impossible: the uniting of psychiatry with medicine and with classical therapeutics. My work was exciting, taking me along a research road where, alone at first, I was now surrounded and joined by many others.

4

Discovery of the antidepressants and mood regulators

Depression—a way of life

Depression is our way of life, and our condition of existence, when we no longer look at the sky, and when we let it fall down on our head. Depression is the mental illness of our time, the most usual, everyday, common and best-known in all the world.

'What is rare,' Kierkegaard wrote, 'is not being in despair; on the contrary, what is rare, the very rarest, is not to be so.' It is because we cannot have everything that we despair. It is also because we cannot keep everything, because our luck runs out. So life only offers us a balance of contrasts, whether it be well-being, pleasure, honour, love, money, or simply the enjoyment of our health and freedom.

Depression can arise, as we shall see, within ourselves or through the influence of circumstances external to us, but always with an eye on what we do not have, or the strange and uncomfortable feeling over what has been taken back from us.

The detachment and lack of interest that sometimes offer easy-going happiness only stand up to depression by borrowing the protection of mysticism or of a calm, sheltering philosophy. But slyly introduced into a skull like a hermit crab into its shell, depression empties it little by little of its willpower, its perceptiveness and its judgement, driving it to anxiety, anguish and despair.

Depression is so general, and so well known, that it is no longer the diagnostic skill of the psychiatrist that detects it, nor even that of the general practitioner, but that of anyone with a little common sense who knows how to recognize in another person the emotions he or she has already suffered through the experience of sorrow, sadness or a setback.

Curiously enough, whilst many psychologists or psychiatrists can claim responsibility for strange, barbaric or little-used names to indicate the varieties of neuroses or psychoses, nobody lays claim to parentage of this word 'depression'. The term was meant to convey the idea of reduction of psychological tension, and of the lowering of brain activity. This is still unconvincing; and if one looks in a dictionary, one realizes that before the middle of the twentieth century, no definition of depression was applied to a mental illness. So should one conclude that depression was not recognized as a pathological entity before the present time?

However, one finds these words: neurasthenia, psychasthenia and, above all, melancholia. For while the terms 'depression' and 'depressive state' did not appear in psychiatry until the twentieth century, melancholia was well known, not only to psychiatrists of the preceding century, but for a very long time, and even before our era.

Depression, melancholia, and manic-depressive psychosis

Melancholia (from the Greek *melanos*, black, and *khole,* bile) is the bile, and the black mood, of the ancients. In Hippocrates one finds numerous references to mania and to melancholia. He identified different forms of melancholia and other mood disorders, but did not recognize the link between the exuberant euphoria of the manic and the depression of the melancholic patient. It was only several centuries later that Aretaeus of Cappadocia established the link between these two states, which often succeed one another in the same patient, with alternating excitation and depression. He also noticed that mania, manic excitation, is most common in young people, and melancholia in older subjects. And so seventeen centuries were to pass with this concept of melancholia as the 'black bile' illness, until the romantic view of melancholia in the nineteenth century came to sweeten this ailment. The melancholia of the poet and visionary is almost pleasant, even cheerful; at least it carries a subtle cachet that distances it from anguish and despair. Esquirol rejected the term 'melancholia', but the association with such frequency in mentally ill patients of excitation and depression gave rise to new terms, such as Baillarger's 'double type' mental disturbance, Falret's 'cyclical' mental illness (which is close to the word 'cyclothymia' used since 1909), and finally the famous manic-depressive psychosis of the German Kraepelin.

All this is only the analysis of a fact now well understood: the existence of successive depression and excitation, alternating for longer or shorter periods, lasting for weeks, months, or even years, which sometimes gets better, or else goes on to a chronic state. In the case of manic excitation, this progresses to chronic mania or delirium, and in the case of a depressive attack, to delirious melancholia. In either case, the spontaneous evolution is liable to be arrested by suicide.

Let us leave these severe forms to return to modern depression, a characteristic of our times. One has tried to label it, to understand it and place it in the context of our everyday lives, for awareness of the pathological nature of some states of sadness and depression dates from our era, where we consider we have a right to expect happiness and well-being from society, and from the State.

If depression is a fact of life, as I have said already, it is not seen as a permanent state of sadness, but alternating with a succession of periods where pleasure and contentment come in their turn; indeed, even noisily manifested euphoria. For depression to be considered a disorder, or illness, the signs that characterize it have to become more prolonged and persistent. This is then *symptomatic depression*. And if this symptomatic depression becomes more severe, it develops into a *depressive syndrome*.

The depressive syndrome

Depression came on one day; a harmful factor acted as a trigger. A bereavement, a separation, a professional disappointment, a simple dispute at home or at work, or even merely a poorly accepted transfer into an older age group (into the thirties, forties or fifties). This triggering factor can, paradoxically, be a favourable event: a success, social promotion, a marriage or an unexpected birth. It can therefore be understood that one speaks of reactive depression, the manner of onset of which is variable, from the *breakdown* that suddenly fells a previously dynamic, optimistic individual, to the masked types, concealed by fatigue, headaches, digestive or cardiac problems, which bounce the depressed patient from one doctor to another, often wasting months consulting non-psychiatric specialists, and thereby further delaying diagnosis and treatment.

So depression has finally developed, with the first and the most important of all the symptoms, asthenia, which the psychiatrists at the beginning of the twentieth century named 'neurasthenia' and 'psychasthenia'. It is a tiredness that can easily be distinguished from organic fatigue, for it does not come on after overworking or a physical illness, it is not helped by rest, it is bad in the morning on awakening and often improves, to disappear by the evening. It goes away under the influence of physical activity, and varies from one day to another, depending on changes in mood. There are also difficulties with sleep, which can mask the onset of depression and which sometimes lead to an addiction to hypnotics (themselves depressants), which is very difficult to cure. It is not complete insomnia, but difficulty in getting off to sleep, associated sometimes with an unconscious fear of sleep or a dread of dreaming. Associated digestive disorders are not uncommon; loss of appetite is common, which sometimes progresses to bulimia, all linked with constipation, belching, hiccups and liverish attacks. Genital disorders are common, and although total amenorrhoea is rare, in women one often sees irregularity of the cycle with painful periods. Sexuality is likewise affected, most often diminished, with impotence and frigidity, but sometimes exaggerated, with nymphomania and satyriasis. While heart palpitations, headaches, dizzy spells and certain subjective feelings are equally common, the major affective symptom of depression remains the sadness of mood.

It is often a revolt against destiny, a cry for help from the family circle, but with remarks like, 'What's the good?', and 'What difference will it make?' There is also anguish, with minor forms of anxiety, worry and anticipation of change; or it may show itself with major crises, with choking, palpitations, and feelings of a lump in the throat. The depressed person's guilt reawakens; brooding over old misdeeds, the flight of time, and a life forever doomed to failure leads to a loss of intellectual effectiveness with memory difficulties, which accentuate the anxiety.

How will the depressed person fare if left untreated? One frequent consequence is alcoholism. 'To drown one's troubles in drink' is not wrong in itself, for alcohol is one of the best chemical anxiolytics, the most active anguish solvent, but only in the first phase of its action; in the second phase, it aggravates the depressive state with the 'hangover', which is in fact a small residual depressive state, which itself gives way to alcohol, thus resulting in escalation. So much so that eventually nobody knows whether they are dealing with an alcoholic depression, alcoholism with depression, or a withdrawal depression.

Following the alcohol, arguments, familial or conjugal disputes, accidents, and social disruptions, the supreme danger comes, which is talked about much more often than it is carried out: suicide. The suicide attempt of the depressed person differs from that of the melancholic, which, as we shall see later, is rarely forgiving. In depression it is more likely to be attempted by the injection of medication or the cutting of veins at the wrist; less risky, but always liable to succeed, perhaps because of lack of attention or indifference from those around who have become accustomed to suicide threats, which are really a 'cry for help'.

In spite of everything, depression can develop for several weeks or months, and, unlike melancholia, which is only amenable to treatment, can respond to external factors that result in an improvement, or even a precarious cure, still leaving in place an unstable personality, liable to relapse with every new conflict.

The type of depression we have just described was formerly treated with kind words, sedatives and suggestion, with some success and many setbacks; but often there was an evolution into much more serious depressive illness, needing more intensive treatment, which often failed.

To understand the drama of evolution of depression following agitation and manic excitation, to glimpse the tragedy that this form of mental illness can bring if left untreated, melancholia must now be described.

Melancholia, the gravest of the depressions

Melancholia is not the most common form of depression, but it is the most spectacular, and the most typical in its manifestations, to the point that it has been described and recognized since history began.

It is really a psychosis, because the patient presents delirious ideas of a distinctive type. Melancholia is said to be an endogenous illness, for, unlike reactive depression, there is no triggering factor. It sometimes comes on dramatically, with a suicide attempt or a crime; sadness, which more often comes on insidiously, appears to be a natural reaction to an unfortunate event. Fatigue and lack of willpower often lead mistakenly to other diagnoses. The cardinal symptom is insomnia—not just difficulty in falling asleep, as in simple depression, but early waking. It is at this stage in the development of the disease that psychiatric examination is essential, to prevent a suicide attempt. I deliberately say psychiatric examination, because the subject's feelings of guilt, the will to self-punishment by suicide, must be sought and brought out. It is these thoughts that allow a simple depression or a depressive asthenia to be distinguished from a true melancholic depression, for which hospitalization is immediately decided upon in all cases, so great is the suicide risk. Firmness in this decision must be rigorous, for makeshift solutions (holidays, rest homes) are ineffective stop-gap measures. At a more advanced stage, the appearance of the melancholic patient provides a diagnostic peg. Weakened, bent over, shoulders dropped, eyes fixed on the ground, these patients drag themselves along rather than walk. On the sorrowful, immobile 'marble' face, the features are drawn downwards and outwards; Schule has described a wrinkle on this face which stretches from the forehead to the root of the nose, and which he has called the 'melancholic omega' because it resembles the Greek letter. The monotonous, drawling, whispering voice has a slow delivery, interspersed with sighs, groans or sobs.

These are the psychological symptoms that dominate the picture, for what strikes one first, right from the initial contact with the patient, is the inhibition and paralysis of thought and movements. Inert, without any will, dumbfounded, restricted to bed or an armchair, the patient is incapable of doing anything: the thought process is slowed, answers to questions often come after a long latent period, but memory and orientation in time and space are preserved. It is at this stage that the melancholic patient's sadness and moral suffering are at their peak. They are fed by the feelings of guilt, which defy all reason: unlike depressed patients, the delirious melancholic confesses to unpardonable crimes, often derisory ('I deserve to die because I did not vote at the last elections') or implausible ('It is my fault that the last terrorist assassination took place').

These delirious self-accusations are felt by the patient as atrociously painful; overcome by evil, living day and night with the call of death—a deserved death—maintained by all kinds of illusions and distorted perceptions, the patient believes that punishment is near.

If all melancholic patients do not commit suicide, this is because at the beginning, paralysed by the illness, they are too inhibited to do so. Instead, care must be taken in the regression phase of melancholia, when the patient is improving; it is at the *end* of the melancholia syndrome that most suicide attempts occur, and one must never relax surveillance of a patient who is getting better, or gives the impression of doing so in order to commit suicide.

The melancholic's suicide can happen suddenly. Sometimes it is the culmination of a meticulously prepared and concealed plan. Sometimes it is what is paradoxically called an 'altruistic suicide': for example, a young melancholic mother kills her children before killing herself. Self-mutilations (Van Gogh cutting off his ear), swallowing pins, or even hunger strikes, are similar forms of suicidal behaviour.

In contradistinction to suicide attempts in depressed patients, the melancholic person's suicide rarely fails: jumping out of a window, drowning, falling in front of a train, and firearms, are all too effective.

Untreated, attacks of melancholy develop over six to twelve months. The older the melancholic patient, and the greater the number of previous relapses, the longer the attack lasts. And so, progressing with time, between periods of remission and long stays in the asylum, the melancholic patient grows older, advancing towards a more or less accentuated mental deterioration, and progressive social isolation.

Faced with the anxiety, anguish and despair of the depressed patient, and the frightening mental distress—as bad as acute physical pain—of the melancholic patient, what can be done to help them?

Treatments for depression up to 1957

We are told that the first case of melancholia was described by Homer in the Iliad. It was Bellerophon, the mythological hero, son of Glaucus and grandson of Sisyphus. He had killed his brother Belleros without knowing it: did his melancholia come on after this murder? We are not told anything about the treatment he was given, whether it was what he asked for, or what was prescribed for him. On the other hand, he was sent on a certain number of missions that kept him fully occupied, from the catching and breaking-in of Pegasus, the winged horse, through the slaying of the monstrous Chimera, up to his victory over the Amazons: he did not have much time to be sorry for himself over his lot, all the more so as the king of Lycia, to thank him, gave him his daughter in marriage, and bequeathed him his throne.

In the Odyssey, the sad hero is Telemachus, in Sparta, who frets while with King Menelaus, and his depression is such that his host orders a feast to distract him. Certainly, wine was drunk, but Helen, who perhaps was not indifferent to the young son of Odysseus, wanted to do even more to dissipate his melancholia:

'She tipped a balm, nepenthe, which gives oblivion to evils, into the wine he was drinking. He who had drunk this mixture could not shed tears for a whole day, even if his mother and father were dead, even if his brother or his much loved son were killed in front of him with a bronze weapon and he saw this with his own eyes. And Zeus's daughter possessed this liquid which was given to her by Polydamna, wife of Thoth in Egypt, a fertile land which produces many balms, some beneficial and some lethal.'

Helen's nepenthe was an opiate elixir, if one looks at its Egyptian origin, cradle of the poppy at that time, and one can say that Telemachus was given a well-suited potion.

We will find closer to our time many other depressed and melancholic patients to whom opium was given and who were submitted to diverse treatments in the last century. But I would have liked very much to have known what the great Esquirol prescribed in the course of treating the depressive episodes of 'Mme de S', whose long-drawn out illness he followed for more than two decades, and whose story he tells us:*

'Mme de S is a young woman married at the age of twenty years to a French civil servant who is working abroad. Mme de S has a strong constitution,' Esquirol tells us. 'She had a baby when she was twenty-one, and six days after the confinement her bed caught fire. She was frightened, cried out, and her milk and lochia dried up; a quarter of an hour later, depression, then mania and rage for two months. She was then in the Ile de France.'

'At the age of twenty-nine, Mme de S had a second attack, provoked by the fall of Batavia where her husband was stationed. Two months of mania, four months of melancholia.'

'At thirty-five years old, another attack caused by the anxiety of a rough sea crossing, and by the despair of her husband's imprisonment, captured by the enemy a long way away. Three months of melancholia.'

'At thirty-nine, in November 1815, fourth attack provoked by her husband being posted abroad, and the death of a close friend. Mania for two months; prolonged melancholia.' [Esquirol does not specify the length.]

This was followed by a fifth episode, the circumstances of which I am going to try to piece together.

The Treaty of 1815 had just given France possession of the colony of Senegal. The government of the Second Restoration had armed four ships at the Isle of Aix to safeguard this reconquest. One of these ships was to carry Julian Desiré de S, appointed Governor of Senegal, and his wife, who was now forty. What piece of bad luck; what provocation of fate, led to the ship *Medusa* being the one selected for Mme de S? What happened next is well known.

---

* From: Esquirol JED (1845) *Mental Maladies* (translated by EK Hunt). Philadelphia: Lea & Blanchard.

Leaving the Isle of Aix on 17 June 1816, the *Medusa*, commanded by the incompetent Duroy de Chaumareyse, a former expatriate, ran aground on the Arguin bank on 2 July, forty leagues from the African coast. A raft twenty metres long and seven metres wide was loaded with 149 passengers, who ended up living together for twelve days. The brig *Argus*, which sighted the raft after these twelve days of death pangs, only took aboard fifteen survivors, the others having been thrown overboard or *eaten by the survivors*. Mme de S and her husband were among the fifteen survivors, and Esquirol tells us:

'Mme de S experienced all the horrors of the shipwreck of the *Medusa*, a shipwreck so unfortunately famous. But Mme de S did not lose her reason.'

Madame de S stood up to the shipwreck, and to the raft; she clutched planks and ropes, perhaps tied to crates and stowage wood. I tried to find her in Géricault's famous painting, but I could only see men. Did she eat human flesh, like the other survivors, and how did she cope with this cannibalism and the other horrors? Very well, Esquirol tells us:

'Mme de S did not take leave of her senses. It is only the follow-ing year that her fifth melancholic attack developed, quite like the previous ones. And she was taken back to France "with sadness, despondency, and gnawing stomach pains".'

At forty-six, Madame de S was to have her sixth attack, and so it goes on. Esquirol takes us through his patient's life, describing for us the melancholic periods 'where the vacant-headed patient believes herself incapable of thought or action; during the attacks she loses a lot of weight, and once the weight loss has become extreme, the end of the attack is not far away.'

Everything happened to this woman—love, war, cannibalism; and also Esquirol, with his blood-letting, his opiate sedatives, cold baths, little calm-ing mixtures; did she perhaps also sit on Leuret's chair? Halfway through the nineteenth century, the French psychiatrist Leuret invented a shaking chair to which the patient was attached, in the middle of a bath filled with water. The rest of the operation can easily be imagined, strangely resem-bling a strategy for extracting confessions by torture. Hydrotherapy, calm-ing potions, opiated or bizarrely concocted with ludicrous ingredients, were the sort of things given to depressed and melancholia patients until the dis-covery of electroconvulsive therapy. Nerve sedatives, bromide, opium in the form of laudanum, kind words, suggestion—all this was made use of; and recreational activities—'distractions'—were also prescribed. Opium and laudanum, which sometimes led to dependency, were mistrusted, and one left cures to the passage of time, eased by thermal treatments.

I have mentioned electroconvulsive therapy, which was a therapeutic revolution in its time, and the excellent results obtained with this method.

Many psychiatrists were hesitant about the treatment, however. Like its inventor, Cerletti, they were worried by the convulsive pantomime and were ready to welcome every other therapeutic procedure favourably. In 1957 they had, with chlorpromazine and the neuroleptics, a chemical treatment for psychoses. They lacked a chemical treatment for depression.

Here again, good luck, as well as the attentive observation of a few scientists, was going to give them what they wanted.

Discovery of the antidepressants

Tricyclic antidepressants

Looking after a depressed patient is a strange task; the exercising of a difficult art. With a raging, mentally disturbed man, you overcome him, and calm him; it is a trial of physical and mental strength with a clear objective. But immobility and sadness do not get better under the influence of a good shaking, or a joyful spectacle. Pushing the bike is not going to make it start. You have to get inside the mechanism, put the scattered parts together, build up a will, a motivation, and show the path, sometimes very narrow, by which the patient will eventually find a way back to activity and, above all, the desire to live.

The neuroleptics, the great psychosis drugs, had brought calm to the tempest, and helped to repair minds that were delirious and carried off by hallucinations and storms of passion. These neuroleptics were found by chance. The first great antidepressant, imipramine (Tofranil), was also discovered thanks to a combination of happy circumstances, the details of which I knew at first hand.

Robert Domenjoz's observations

In 1955, while studying the actions of aromatic essences and perfumes on the central nervous system, I found that oil of clove, which is an aromatic phenol, could be chemically modified and converted into a substance with considerable hypnotic power. I had even succeeded, with Dr Bernard Sadoun and Dr Boureau, in putting patients to sleep with this substance to carry out narcoanalyses and electroconvulsive therapy under anaesthesia, about which I will speak later. A difficulty cropped up when it came to the intravenous injection of the drug, because it was not soluble in water and a solvent had to be found that would not be irritant to the veins. The problem of refining this solvent had interested the Geigy laboratory in Basle, who were studying the development of an injectable form with me. For this study I was in touch with the Geigy scientific management, and particularly with the chemists Stoll and Litvan, and especially with Robert Domenjoz, the director of pharmacological research.

Domenjoz, a sharp, cultured man, a well-informed clinician and a wise pharmacologist, already had some top-quality work to his credit. A contemporary and colleague of Paul Muller, with whom he had studied the insecticidal properties of DDT, it was he who also demonstrated the anti-inflammatory activity of phenylbutazone (Butazolidine), which is still one of the most powerful antirheumatic agents known. Immediately after the discovery of the neuroleptics and chlorpromazine, Domenjoz and the Geigy laboratory devoted a large part of their research activities to the study of nervous system drugs, principally a series of chemical molecules related to Spécia's chlorpromazine. Amongst the chemical series prepared were products which, like chlorpromazine, had a tricyclic structure (with three rings).

Pharmacological studies of these products had shown that they were quite different from the neuroleptics, having no antihistaminic activity and leading to no sedation in normal or agitated animals. They did not cause cataplexy, that stiff attitude, almost paralytic, which was seen in animals treated with chlorpromazine. Quite the contrary: cataplexy provoked by chlorpromazine could be suppressed by administration of these tricyclic compounds, and one of them, imipramine, was particularly active in this respect. It is for this reason, albeit with a certain hesitancy, that Robert Domenjoz had suggested imipramine to a few psychiatrists to try out in mentally ill patients. At that time the whole orientation of the clinical trials on psychotropic drugs was directed towards treatment of the major psychoses with agitation and ravings. Imipramine, Geigy's tricyclic drug, proved much less active than chlorpromazine in these cases, and the product was about to be abandoned after fruitless trials by Swiss and German psychiatrists, who preferred chlorpromazine. And then, one day, a certain Roland Kuhn entered the picture.

The development of imipramine

Robert Domenjoz often came to Paris. One winter morning in 1957 I had gone to meet him at the Gare de l'Est, and after coffee in a bar, we went back to Sainte-Anne.

We had to prepare the text of a scientific communication that was to appear in a special issue of the German journal *Der Anaesthesist*. In it we recounted the story of the discovery of intravenous anaesthesia with clove, which we had perfected with a product that was to become the front runner of a new class of non-barbiturate intravenous anaesthetics. At the end of our labours, Robert Domenjoz took out from his attaché case a small bottle on which was stuck a label bearing the number G22355, and which contained some small, white tablets.

'I've already spoken to you,' he said, 'about our trials with the tricyclics, looking for new neuroleptics analogous to Largactil. These products turned out to be a good deal less active than chlorpromazine. Our psychiatrists in Zürich and Basle, and other German clinicians, have given up using them after negative trials; however, I have a problem to solve. I gave one of these products to a psychiatrist who works in a small cantonal hospital. I know him well, he is a conscientious man, and a scrupulous observer whose intuition and clinical experience I have often made use of for other drugs. Now, contrary to the big customers, he is insistent that clinical experiments should continue with one of the tricyclics, which is imipramine and which we have given the name Tofranil.'

Domenjoz was perplexed and embarrassed: the Geigy medical management wanted to tidy the product away in the 'forgotten products' cupboard, but he himself was uncertain.

'Roland Kuhn has never misled me, and this time, he is insistent; he persists. He states he has obtained spectacular results in depressions. It appears that the product must be administered for several weeks to obtain an effect quite different from that of the neuroleptics, for, according to him, the drug only works in depression. He had even achieved cures in some cases of severe melancholia without needing to resort to electroconvulsion.'

Robert Domenjoz had such confidence in the clinical intuition of Roland Kuhn that he begged me to ask Jean Delay to try the product at Sainte-Anne. As far as I was concerned, I did not know Roland Kuhn, but I knew that if Domenjoz insisted on this point, I could trust him. A few moments after his request, we were in Jean Delay's study with Pierre Deniker, and after repeating to them what he had told me, it was agreed to start experiments in the department.

This is how one of the first bottles of Tofranil arrived at Sainte-Anne for experiments that were to last several months and which did not immediately turn out happily. For the tricyclics, as they were later to be called, have the remarkable property of altering and correcting depressive disturbances of mood, but in some cases, their effects can go further than intended and change the morose mood into euphoria, which could go as far as manic excitation. In the course of this transfer from one extreme to the other, the patient must be constantly supervised, for at that time there can be a risk of suicide.

Although remarkably effective, imipramine, which remains the front runner of the tricyclic antidepressants, did not immediately give Deniker satisfactory results. The treatment needed to be codified, each case analysed, and the results collated. In other university hospital centres experiments were being pursued and positive results were multiplying, but it can be said that it was thanks to Roland Kuhn's persistence and Robert Domenjoz's enlightened tenacity that imipramine became established as the first chemotherapy for melancholia and the depressions, capable in a large number of cases of replacing electroconvulsive therapy.

In September 1957 Roland Kuhn published the results of his experiments with imipramine in a Swiss medical journal; it was the first work on one of the two types of antidepressants: the tricyclic antidepressants.

Thanks to simultaneous observations by a group of biochemists and a remarkable American psychiatrist, a second type of true antidepressant was to be discovered in the same year, 1957: the inhibitors of monoamine oxidase, signified by the letters MAOI.

The MAOIs

After the discovery of the neuroleptics, chlorpromazine and reserpine, a discovery due in large measure to good luck, the laboratory teams turned their attention to trying to understand how these drugs worked. They could not elucidate the origin of psychoses and mental illness, but they tried to understand the mechanism of action of these drugs that cured them: where did they act, and what disruptions did they produce in the blood and the fluids that bathe our tissues and brain?

Let us say right away that the studies on chlorpromazine (Largactil) did not give conclusive results; in contrast reserpine (Serpasil), whose neuroleptic activity had been discovered by Nathan S. Kline, showed itself to be a research tool of particular interest to the biochemists. They had found that the administration of reserpine to the rabbit, and to all mammals (rats, mice, etc.) caused almost complete disappearance of the monoamines in the brains of these animals.

I have spoken of these substances found in the brain called neurotransmitters, because it is thanks to them that our nervous system functions and transmits messages. These neurotransmitters are chemical substances that are also called monoamines, and which play an essential role.

Thus animals injected with reserpine, and which were calm, indeed even exhausted and depressed, no longer had monoamines in the brain. From there to conclude that diminution in monoamines (abbreviated MA) in the brain led to calm and sedation took only one step. But the converse remained to be proved: to show that excess of MA would cause excitation and agitation. For this, it was necessary to paralyse the oxidase enzyme that destroys MA; this was achieved using a monoamine oxidase inhibitor (MAOI).

In other words, with an MAOI one could reverse the depressive effect of reserpine, by preventing the brain from losing its monoamines. Therefore, the MAOIs must be antidepressants.

I hope my reasoning has been followed, because it explains the unique example of a rational discovery of a brain drug; not a chance finding, but the result of scientific deduction. And now, we will see how this was translated into practice.

Nathan S. Kline, a psychiatrist unlike others

I think my friend Nathan Kline would not wish me to describe him as 'a psychiatrist unlike others'. For me, this is a compliment, for the great discoveries he has made show that his curiosity, his imagination and the genius of his powers of association are unrivalled. The speed of his judgement is only equalled by his talent to exercise it in practice, and the value of his hypotheses always call for the most attentive examination.

I have already recounted how Kline, at Rockland State Hospital, starting from the observation of cardiac patients depressed by reserpine, came to use the drug to treat the excitation of acute psychosis and of raving delirium. It is on this neuroleptic depressive action of reserpine that Brodie and his collaborators were working. When they used MAOIs to enliven and reawaken animals immobilized or stupefied by reserpine, Kline wanted to know which these MAOIs were, and whether these chemical products had yet been used in therapeutics. The MAOIs used by Brodie and his collaborators were generally the 'hydrazides'—substances not free from toxicity, but Kline knew that one of them was widely used in the treatment of tuberculosis; this was isoniazid (isonicotinic acid hydrazide), manufactured, with the trade name Rimifon, by the Hoffmann–La Roche laboratory in Basle. Kline remembered that in the treatment of tuberculosis with isoniazid, all observers had been struck by the extraordinary improvement in the general condition of the patients who, even before the Koch's bacilli had disappeared from the lesions, exhibited euphoria, improved appetite, and even in some cases a degree of excitation which had sometimes necessitated the administration of sedatives.

Tuberculosis patients excited by isoniazid, animals depressed by reserpine and revived by products analogous to isoniazid: right away Kline wanted to know if isoniazid was an MAOI, and as this was actually the case, he tried isoniazid and immediately another hydrazide, iproniazid (Marsilid), which allowed him to successfully treat depressions and severe melancholias.

Thus, helped by the remarkable biochemical study by Brodie, and the marketing by Hoffmann–La Roche of an easy-to-handle MAOI, Kline succeeded in less than four years in achieving the impressive double of finding one of the first two neuroleptics and one of the first two antidepressants.

The tricyclics and the MAOIs

Between imipramine and Kuhn's tricyclics, and Kline's iproniazid and the MAOIs, there was no problem in deciding which of these two types of antidepressants to choose, for quickly each found its place in a therapeutic line-up allowing the two categories of depression to be treated selectively.

So, broadly speaking, one could say: the frank melancholia syndrome, with mental distress, anguish, inhibition, thoughts of incurability, uselessness and suicide, recovered with tricyclics and in particular imipramine. To put it another way, all conditions calling for electroconvulsive therapy, principally the melancholias, could be treated with imipramine under medical supervision, in the clinic or in hospital. Patients in the other category, with simple depression, whether exogenous or reactive, with physical or mental asthenia, anxiety, despondency or sexual impotence, recovered with MAOIs and iproniazid, given orally on an out-patient basis.

In practice, this oversimplified distinction is now of little value, because many depressions are also treated with tricyclics such as imipramine. Since Kuhn's and Kline's discoveries, in each of the two groups of products many other derivatives have been found that are effective in the different varieties of depression. It must be understood, however, that the handling of antidepressants, like that of neuroleptics, is very delicate and that it must be completely under the control of specialist doctors accustomed to using these products, which must not, in principle, be given together, or administered with alcohol or certain foodstuffs. For example, patients taking MAOI drugs must avoid cheese, as there is a risk of setting off an arterial hypertensive crisis, which could be fatal.

Mood regulators

Depression and melancholia well treated with tricyclics or MAOIs most often do not require electroconvulsive therapy; but just as electroconvulsive therapy does not prevent recurrences in patients subject to relapses, so antidepressants do not guarantee a permanent cure in patients prone to recurrent depressive attacks.

Alternation, the more or less closely following succession of signs of uncontrolled mental excitation and deep depression, represents one of the most disruptive mental disturbances for the individual; these conditions are called 'mood disorders'. This term covers the illness sometimes still known as cyclothymia or manic-depressive psychosis. The psychopharmacological discoveries made it possible to treat the excitation phase effectively with neuroleptics, and the depressive phase with antidepressants. However, an ideal therapy would achieve stabilization of these disorders, these derangements of mood, and this was the object of the third great discovery—that of the mood regulators.

Dr Gustin's lithium salts

I remember from my childhood, and so perhaps will some of you, Dr Gustin's lithium salts. Waterproof metal boxes could be purchased in pharmacies containing sachets of a powder that had to be mixed with water to produce a fizzy drink. In the box, beside the sachets, was a little cardboard funnel, which had to be unfolded and put in the neck of a bottle previously filled with water. The powder in a sachet was tipped through the funnel, and the bottle was quickly re-corked and shaken up once or twice. The powder was seen dissolving with an effervescence that sometimes made the cork shoot out of the bottle if it had not been pushed in hard enough. The beverage thus prepared was called a 'lithium drink'; it was drunk on its own or mixed with wine. The leaflet with the box said it was a sovereign remedy for gout and urinary stones, that the drink was hygienic and dietetic, and that it could be taken generally.

Certainly in those days when we did not have good carbonated mineral water, the tangy flavour of Dr Gustin's lithium salts was appreciated. The indications on the leaflet relied on the fact that lithium salts dissolve urinary stones formed by uric acid (urates). These salts included lithium oxide, also known as 'lithia'.

Lithium, a forgotten metal

Who discovered this lithium, which is present in nearly all mineral water springs? It is said that in the days of antiquity the water from certain springs cured patients with delirium, especially the noisy ones. It would be interesting now to identify these springs and to measure the lithium salt or lithia levels. More recently, in Henderson and Gillespie's *Textbook of Psychiatry* there is a list of alkaline water springs in Cornwall, Scotland, and Wales that cured mania. But there was nothing to suggest the significance of this metal, unknown as such until 1817, when it was identified by the Swedish chemist Arfvedson. His master, the famous Baron Johan Jakob Berzelius, to whom we owe our symbolic chemical nomenclature, named the new element 'lithium', and marvelled at its unique characteristics. Almost certainly if the alchemists had known of lithium, they would have talked about it. I imagine Paracelsus discovering, with amazed delight, the lightest of all the solid elements, the hardest of the alkali metals, the substance with the greatest specific heat, the greatest stability with fluorine, and liberating the greatest amount of energy when combining with water ...

At the end of the nineteenth century the discovery that lithium oxide dissolved urates introduced this element into therapeutics for gout and renal lithiasis. In 1927 another discovery was made. Bromides were in fashion, and it was found that lithium bromide is the most hypnotic of the bromides. It was used in epilepsy, but cardiac and renal damage was encountered.

Apart from the non-toxic lithium salts, lithium was to be forgotten until 1949.

From Australia to Denmark via France

It was the Australian John Cade who first used lithium in psychiatry, in 1949. I have not been able to find out exactly why he first tried lithium on guinea pigs. It seems he wanted to eliminate or reduce the toxicity of urea, and he had soluble lithium urate prepared, which he tried on the guinea pigs. He was surprised to see that the animals appeared conscious but immobile, as if in a state of lethargy, and that although not asleep they remained still and did not respond to stimuli. It was then that he thought of using lithium in manic excitation with agitation, but for this he had lithium carbonate made. At the end of a year, Cade had gathered fifty observations on manic excitation cured with lithium carbonate. But regrettably there were a few mishaps, and even one unexplained death.

John Cade was a little-known psychiatrist, and Australia was remote from the centres of research in Europe and America. Little attention was paid to his work, which was published in an Australian medical journal. However, in 1951, at the annual Congress of French-Speaking Psychiatrists and Neurologists, Despinoy and de Romeuf reported their 'use of lithium salts in psychiatry'. They, too, had good results in manic-depressive psychoses. In spite of this, lithium salts were more or less abandoned because of unexplained failures and toxic complications, which seemed to be unpredictable and serious. Furthermore, lithium and its salts were available to anybody, and the pharmaceutical companies were much more interested in developing new neuroleptic and antidepressant molecules that they could patent. Nevertheless, a Danish psychiatrist became interested in lithium; and it was the determined and persevering work of Mogens Schou, rather than the original reports by John Cade, that ensured the development of this strange metal in psychiatric therapeutics.

The stubbornness of Mogens Schou

It was beginning to get ridiculous. Since 1955, at all therapeutic congresses, seminars and meetings where psychiatrists gathered to talk about new chemotherapies for psychoses, a young, blond doctor would stand up and talk in a calm, quiet way about lithium. Sometimes, when allowed, he presented a paper or gave an account of results, but usually he only joined in the discussion because he was prevented from repeating what was regarded as a lot of chatter that was turning into an obsession. In spite of this, Mogens Schou was not offended. Tirelessly, he repeated that in the lithium salts it was the lithium that was active, and that the effectiveness and harmlessness of the product was in direct proportion to the level of lithium in the blood.

'If you do not give enough,' he said, 'this is no use. If you give too much, you may have serious and even fatal complications.'

I have mentioned that I met Schou for the first time at Aarhus in 1956, and that at the neurochemistry congress banquet where we ate sweetened chicken, he had spoken to me about lithium. I often came across Schou again, between 1956 and 1968, in psychiatry congresses, neuropsychopharmacology Collegium meetings, and therapeutic colloquia; each time, his insistence and obstinacy surprised and even annoyed us. It was almost forgotten that he was an excellent psychiatrist and that while he used lithium, he also, like everybody else, prescribed the other psychotropic drugs. For him it was even a roundabout way of bringing up lithium when he was comparing its effects with other antidepressants.

I have recorded that at the Rome congress in 1958, where more than fifty participants reported their results obtained with imipramine and the MAOIs, there was also a paper from Schou on lithium that went quite unnoticed.

Then, one day Schou succeeded in convincing the other Danish psychiatrists: first his chief, Strömgren, and then his colleagues Baastrup and Hartigan; and little by little the number of scientific reports published on this topic grew. From 1959 until 1963, there were fifteen publications on lithium; from 1964 to 1968, thirty. In 1975 there were more than three thousand reports, notes and papers on lithium's extraordinary capacity to be both a curative and a preventive treatment for mood disorders.

Lithium, a mood regulator

Mood is an attitude of mind that determines the character of the moment, both as regards what is stable and permanent, and also what is capricious, whimsical and impulsive. In the middle of this ever-changing scene, reason must prevail, and for me, this is what controls the mood; and so, when reason is no longer there, resort must be made to lithium.

I have just written this like a witticism, but even so I feel comfortable with this definition of lithium as a 'mood regulator'.

Lithium regulates the mood of our inner 'self' by becoming integrated with our psychological personality. It is characterized by its double action, at the same time correcting psychological and mental excitation, whilst preventing expansive and depressive derangements of mood. It is in its preventive role against relapses of mania and depression that lithium is unique. It has truly made it possible to distinguish a new class of drugs—that of the 'psychological function regulators'.

Its distinctive action is neither closely nor distantly like any other psychotropic drug. With lithium there are no more 'sudden mood changes', no more exuberant behaviour or extreme depression, no more expansiveness or morbid regression; instead, there is equilibrium and equanimity. For this, two or three lithium carbonate tablets or two or three ampoules of lithium gluconate are needed daily; but caution—before starting treatment, a careful assessment must be made of the kidneys, the heart, the thyroid and the nervous system, since lithium is toxic for all these organs if its level in the blood rises above a certain threshold. For this reason, the lithaemia (level of lithium in the blood) must be measured every eight days at the beginning of treatment, and every month when the effective dose has been reached.

The start of lithium treatment must be closely controlled by the doctor to detect tremors, digestive upsets, urinary symptoms and, above all, overdosage, which can be fatal. Gradually, treatment becomes stabilized at a steady daily dosage with regular administration of the effective dose.

When lithium is prescribed as a preventive, to avoid the recurrence of manic-depressive attacks, the duration of treatment is indeterminate. It may stretch over many years. Stopping medication or substitution of another product in place of lithium has been seen to be associated with an increased percentage of relapses. So treatment can only be left off if lithium becomes contraindicated.

Thus Schou's perseverance made possible the introduction into psychiatric therapeutics of a simple chemical substance that has helped millions of depressed people in the world through a still unknown mechanism, for none of the hypotheses on the mechanism of action of lithium has ever been verified.

Nowadays, Schou is invited to all the scientific meetings on mood disorders and depressions; he is now a welcome speaker, perhaps partly as an apology for the long indifference to his words.

If you are depressed . . .

If you become depressed, read the *Works and Days* of Hesiod. Choose the chapter on the Golden Age, and dream:

> 'Humans lived then like the gods, with their heart free of worries, far from work and pain. Sad old age did not come to them, and retaining the vigour of their feet and hands throughout their life, they savoured joy in feasts, sheltered from all evil. They died as if going off to sleep, overcome with drowsiness. Everything good was theirs. The fertile land offered them abundant food, which they enjoyed as they wished.'

When the dream draws to an end in the reading, nostalgia for the impossible will overcome you: this Golden Age must be cast into the future, instead of going back to the beginning of time. If everything upsets you, do not take refuge in scepticism and doubt. Search your surroundings, analyse your so-called destitution, and the wounds in your soul . . . but now I am dreaming too. Everybody is not Kierkegaard to write a *Treatise on Despair*, or St Augustine to bare his soul in *Confessions*, and still less Robert Burton to compile the *Anatomy of Melancholy*. In this book, published in 1621 and considered to be the greatest medical treatise ever written by a layman, Robert Burton declares: 'If other men derive their knowledge from books, I get mine from the habit of melancholy.'

So, if you are melancholic, you will know everything. First, you will learn that you are not alone. There are more than a hundred million depressed people in the world, and this number grows steadily. Here is some more information: in a population of a thousand people, one hundred and fifty depressed patients do not consult any doctor, look after themselves and get better on their own; twelve will go to see a general practitioner; and only two a psychiatrist. It should be appreciated that up to half of the patients who consult are not suffering from any illness, and it is correct to think that they have gone to see the doctor because they were depressed. Finally, in a population of ten thousand people, one suicide, one compulsory admission, and seven hospitalizations for depression can be expected.

These statistics are the result of epidemiological surveys, and it is interesting to ask people what they think about depression.

Out of all the individuals questioned, 100% think that everybody in the world has had one depression in their life; 92% think that to be depressed is not just to be unhappy; 83% prefer to handle the problem of their depression by themselves rather than go to a psychiatrist; 82% prefer the help of a friend to that of a doctor; and 93% think that a cure is a matter of willpower.

From these answers, one can see the extent to which public opinion can adopt ready-made ideas that unfortunately do not take account (and for a very good reason) of the specificity of every depression. This is why, if it is necessary and desirable that the greatest number of depressive states should be treated by general physicians, these doctors should be better prepared to respond to the demand in this field. Non-psychiatrist doctors often miss cases of serious melancholia, conjuring up an illness said to be neurovegetative or organic; or, in contrast, labelling a mild depressive state as an anxiety neurosis. From one practitioner to another, the concept of depression varies. One Swiss psychiatric doctor, Dr Paul Kielholz of Basle, has drawn up a list of simple questions that enable a confirmed depressive state to be identified. Here is this questionnaire:

1   Do you still enjoy anything?
2   Do you have difficulty making decisions?
3   Are you still interested in anything?
4   Do you tend to get lost in morose ruminations?
5   Do you complain of no longer finding any meaning in your life?
6   Do you feel tired, without relief?
7   Do you sleep badly?
8   Do you have pain or a heavy feeling in your chest?
9   Do you lack appetite, and have you lost weight?
10   Do you have difficulties in sexual relations?

If you answer 'no' to questions 1 and 3, and 'yes' to all the others, you are certainly depressed; but the diagnosis is not just made with this questionnaire, for many other considerations should be taken into account: difficulty in concentration, the nature of the insomnia, remorse, irritability ... this is why it is better to consult a good psychiatrist. You should have no fear of a good psychiatrist, who is always reassuring. The psychiatrist will ask you, 'When did the trouble start?'

You yourself will ask, 'How long is it going to last?'

The psychiatrist will reply that this depends on the way you respond to treatment. You will ask what treatment you are going to receive, and whether psychotherapy will be needed. The answer will be that medication will probably work on its own, but it must be continued for a certain time. When you are cured—because you have been told that you are—you will ask, 'And if it comes back?'

'We'll have to see . . .'

But let us stop this facile recital, the reality is more testing than my prose suggests, and more complex than my sentences indicate. I would like to reassure you without deceiving you and without diminishing your vigilance. Yes, depression and melancholia can now be cared for and cured without Pinel's red-hot cautery, without Leuret's shaking chair in iced water, and without stagnating for months in the asylum. Thanks to the discovery of the antidepressants, you can stand up to the anguish of the world, brought into your home by the press, radio and television. Finally, if your breakdown is resistant to tricyclics and the MAOIs, as happens with fifteen per cent of depressed patients, you will still have the opportunity to undergo King Arthur's treatment.

King Arthur and electronarcosis

King Arthur, alias Torquemada, was in fact Claude B, whom I had had to admit to hospital one morning at Sainte-Anne after he had broken a desk lamp on the hospital chief physician's head. I described at the beginning of this book the manic-depressive attack that this colleague experienced in the 1950s.

He was nicknamed Torquemada when he was exuberant, in memory of the crisis in which he had accused everybody of sorcery; and as he was a Breton from Quimper, tall and bearded, and often sententious, he was also called King Arthur.

I had lost sight of King Arthur at the end of my residency job; I knew that after ups and downs his health had improved and that he practised medicine in Brittany. By chance a holiday led to my meeting him again in Cornouaille, in South Finistère, in the port of Bénodet, a few years ago. Dressed in elegantly washed-out trousers and sailor's smock, still tall, slim and bearded, King Arthur was mooring his boat and gathering his sails. The reunion was warm and almost moving. We had to meet again and talk. There was so much to say. We decided on a fishing expedition.

We left the Coq buoy at dawn, and the *Picoteux* sailed out through the Odet estuary. She is a big Breton fibreglass boat; a little bulbous but stable and good for fishing. The mainsail and jib pull us on towards the open sea, and already the sun is slipping up like the quarter of an orange at the tip of the Trévignon point. We are bound for the Glénans islands to put out some prawn pots on the shoals, and will be fishing for a few Norway pout with long lines. I am at the helm while King Arthur gets the bait ready for the lines and puts handfuls of sardine heads into the neck of the pots.

'My word! It's better here than the rue de la Perche!'

King Arthur is standing upright and filling his lungs with fresh air. In the rue de la Perche was a private psychiatric clinic where he had undergone many treatments.

'Do you still remember the rue de la Perche?'

He remembered everything, did King Arthur. His episode with Dr Abely, his reading of the *Malleus Maleficarum*, which had put the delirium concerned with the destruction of heretics into his head, and his numerous bouts of depression, alternating with manic excitation.

'It was Father Lampin who gave me the electric convulsion treatments, and sometimes little Bodard, when he was absent. The first thing I saw when I came out from my haze was her rounded buttocks squeezed into her narrow skirt.'

How many electroconvulsive treatments did King Arthur have? Dozens, no doubt.

'And then one day, the new drugs were tried. First Tofranil, but this turned my mood upside down . . .'

He was calmed down with neuroleptics, treated again with tricyclic antidepressants, then moved on to MAOI antidepressants. He improved for a time, then the problem came back, sometimes depression, sometimes the beginnings of excitation, quickly arrested with powerful sedatives. Years passed, not too good or too bad, and then one day the illness returned, this time with great despair, abysmal depression, complete darkness.

'They did everything for me, at the rue de la Perche. They wanted to get to the bottom of everything. First it was certain: it all came from my mother; my 'manic depression' was the prototype of the genetically transmitted illness, the finest example known of a psychiatric affective disorder with Mendelian inheritance. Yes, sir! By dominant transmission through the X chromosome. Then it was explained to me that the Marsilid they were giving me was no longer active, because in me the MAOIs did not increase the serotonin in my brain sufficiently. And as Tofranil no longer worked either, it proved that the tricyclic antidepressants could no longer prevent the neurotransmitter uptake at the level of the synaptic junction.'

King Arthur had fully understood everything they had told him at the rue de la Perche clinic. The genetics of his inherited illness, like most straightforward depressions, had been explained to him because he was a doctor. It was also explained to him how the two classes of antidepressants worked and why they did not work in his case. King Arthur was one of the minority of depressed patients who cease to respond to antidepressants.

King Arthur began to be severely depressed, with suicidal thoughts. He felt lost within his poor head, so often bounced from one depression to another, and one manic crisis to another; all the more lost because this time he refused shock treatment, the gag, the electrodes on his temples, and the 'convulsive pantomime' which he had not only seen in others, but had had to undergo himself in the past. The show was over, the impossible quest for the Grail and the feasts at the Round Table have come to an end. It was to be the death of King Arthur; but the enchanter Merlin was still watching over him.

First he reassured him, electroconvulsive therapy was quite finished: now there was *electronarcosis*.

Very nicely, you are laid on a comfortable bed, and an anaesthetist gently puts a needle into a vein at the fold of the elbow. Slowly, very slowly, a little thiopentone sodium (Pentothal) is injected, which sends you pleasantly off to sleep, and when you are slumbering, unconscious, sometimes carried away by a lovely dream, the anaesthetist injects something else through the same needle. This time it is some curare, but a mild formulation, with a quick, short action. The muscles immediately relax, the body goes slack and limp, and it is then that the electrodes are placed on the temples of the sleeping patient and an electric current is passed. It is the same apparatus, the same current at the same strength, but it is no longer the same patient, tensed, anxious and conscious. The current crosses a sleeping brain, and the wave of convulsion passes through a relaxed, limp body whose muscles will only show a slight quivering. In front of the slightly opened lips the anaesthetist will hold a plastic mask with an oxygen respirator which will revive the respiration depressed by the curare; and gradually the patient will regain consciousness, hardly dispelled by the Pentothal, and strength, so little affected by the curare.

The 'drama' of electroconvulsive therapy had been replaced by 'interludes' of electronarcosis. The subject and the scenery are much the same, a few props have simply been added; but the production has been thought through again and studied, and this makes all the difference for the audience, even though the moral of the play is unchanged. In the treatment of depression it is no longer a tragic sequence, but rather a diversionary interlude.

Electronarcosis lifted King Arthur out of the abyss of his melancholia, refractory to antidepressants, and it will save many more mentally ill patients. Ugo Cerletti remains responsible for thousands of cures with this improved electroconvulsive therapy, disguised and made less alarming, now known as electronarcosis.

'It was at the end of my second course of electronarcosis that I was given lithium. I was one of the first to take it, and for the last eight years, my mood has been like the sea this morning!'

A land breeze carried us towards the open sea, smoothing the water which barely rippled. The sun was now climbing over the Glénans. We put out our pots and caught some rockling and Norway pout. At midday, after anchoring at the Moutons, we had lunch on the north shore of the island. King Arthur showed me his bottle of lithium tablets.

'My gree gree!'

I had never seen him so calm and serene. This was certainly helped by the relaxation of this day's fishing, the peaceful silence of the sea, and the shared pleasure of an old friendship. I also knew, though, that an effective mediator was controlling King Arthur's inner peace. In his blood there was circulating a light metal which intervened at every moment to offer its good offices. The lithium which permeated my friend's 'humours' also regulated his 'mood' like a pendulum or a well-balanced rudder. And all this was not so bad, after the storms.

So, if you are depressed, no more fear or trembling; think of King Arthur, of the help and support of the psychiatrist and of modern psychopharmacology, which discovered how to make drugs acting against despondency, anguish and anxiety. Even if the product best suited for your condition is not found right away, do not be frightened of the heroic and always worthwhile treatment of electronarcosis, and know that lithium will readjust your mood long-term.

But if you are merely sad and despondent, if your ideas, which you think are black, are only grey, you will not need King Arthur's treatments, and you will just be prescribed a few tranquillizers.

5
Discovery of the tranquillizers

What is a tranquillizer?

The Pope and the tranquillizers

Emilio Trabucchi, as always, had done things very well for the first Congress of the CINP in Rome. Scientific meetings in the new EUR buildings, receptions at the Castel Sant' Angelo, at the Borghese palace, in the gardens of the Villa d'Este, and finally, an audience with the Pope in his residence at Castel Gandolfo.

We waited for a long time in a large room in the central building. The number of psychiatrists and pharmacologists had been limited, for the audience room at the Pope's summer residence was not very big and the pontiff was already very ill. It was unbearably hot in this room, of which we only occupied a part of the floor. Half of the room was raised as a platform which ran from one wall to the other, with a recess with two windows and two doors facing one another.

The two doors opened and two Swiss Guards positioned themselves on either side of a third central door, through which the Pope entered, followed by a few prelates.

Eugenio Pacelli, who was to die exactly one month later, was eighty-two years old. He had always been thin, and his emaciated, pale face surprised nobody. In spite of the extreme heat in the audience room, he was wearing a woollen jacket on top of his white cassock, and I also noticed that he had a kind of knitted tie covering his neck. Trabucchi climbed the two steps that led onto the platform, bowed to kiss the Fisherman's Ring, and, quite at ease, gave the names of the nationalities of the psychopharmacologists present and the theme of the congress that had brought us together in Rome. Briefly, he set out the progress made in psychiatric therapeutics in the last five years, and justified the existence of a new discipline whose methods and aims he explained.

Pius XII had listened to Trabucchi standing up, but meantime an armchair had been brought on to the platform, and he sat on it to read us a kind of homily written like a lecture, full of directives, instructions and formal orders. The beginning was tedious enough, for the compiler of the text, to show he understood the question well, explained what psychopharmacology was; but I awaited with curiosity the recommendations at the end of the speech, which concerned us directly. Pius XII, with whose political attitudes in the course of the Second World War there was not always general agreement, was an enquiring mind who took upon himself the task of clarifying the Christian doctrine as it faced the modern world. And so, on philosophical and scientific levels, he had taken up clear positions, and if I did not like his condemnation of Freudianism, at least the dialectic used had interested me. I also waited for the final instruction with interest.

Having recognized that the use of psychotropic drugs had made it possible to reduce the length of time spent in hospital by patients suffering from severe psychoses significantly, and to humanize the treatment and the conditions for the mentally ill, Pius XII began to talk of the use of tranquillizers to soothe the sufferings of the soul; and there, doubts came to assail him.

'Life', he said, 'every day brings burdens and problems which must be confronted with lucidity, and resolved with Christian faith and wisdom. Now, it is to retreat before stress, and to reject one's responsibilities to ask a drug to create indifference and oblivion in the face of one's duties; this is a fatal renunciation which can only end in compromises and failure. An anxiety must take care of itself, mobilizing its strength to draw up plans and bring realistic behaviour to a successful conclusion, whereby the Christian derives something from faith, hope and charity.'

I had been distracted at the end of the speech because the heat of the room was having repercussions. Uncomfortable congress members, taken ill, had been evacuated as discreetly as possible, but this had caused a stir at the back of the room. Unperturbed, Pius XII went on with his harangue. The tranquillizers had interested him but left him puzzled; he saw in them mysterious remedies about which little was yet known concerning either their use or the significance of their effects. The psychotropes that caused hallucinations, like LSD, he had rejected because they undermined human dignity: as for the neuroleptics (the Americans' 'major tranquillizers'), he could but accept them as essential medicines; and as regards the tranquillizers that were becoming distributed throughout the world, not enough time had yet gone by to make a judgement; but he sensed there, in pills and tablets, a power that made the doctor almost into a sorcerer. Between his words one could detect his fears and apprehensions. Was it to see doctors acquire greater power, and patients lose what remained of their mental autonomy?

The homily ended with a mild hubbub at the back of the room where other people, overcome by the heat, were indicating their intention to leave. The Pope finally rose to give his benediction, and I saw that he still had a great presence. A few days afterwards, he was to start a bout of hiccups, which persisted until his death a month later.

When we left the palace, big drops of rain began to fall and a storm broke out over Lake Albano, which fills the site of an ancient crater. On the slopes surrounding the lake, vineyards under trees rose in terraces. In the distance, cypresses and parasol pines fringed the curves of hills thrown up millions of years earlier from the inferno of molten magma. And on the edge of this extinct volcano, in his sumptuous and peaceful palace, in the autumn in this Roman countryside, a fragile man, in precarious health, but whose authority rules over millions of souls, had been willing to speak to us of his own scruples, paradoxically worried and agitated by tranquillizers.

What is a tranquillizer?

On this day in September 1958, tranquillizers, their use and perhaps their abuse, were preoccupying the Pope. What were these tranquillizers? What was their place amongst the great psychosis drugs (neuroleptics) and the drugs for depression and melancholia (antidepressants)?

At the beginning of the twentieth century such drugs were called painkillers, sedatives and antispasmodics. They were to modify the functional activity of an organ or system, for it was especially the heart and the nerves that were involved. The mind, the psyche, was a matter for the sphere of common sense, and a friendly word from a close friend or priest. The preoccupations of life, anguish and anxiety, found their solution in people's attitude towards resolving these problems. However, with some reactions it was found that the mind influenced the body and its systems, sending them pointless impulses and setting up harmful disturbances. Family doctors, who knew about the life and history of their patients, set themselves, in their advice, to play down the importance of situations, and explain the conflicts. When they did not succeed with kind words, they prescribed remedies; first herbal tea—sage, camomile—then bromides, small doses of hypnotics, Crataegus, or valerian mixed with henbane. Some famous doctors had marketed formulas that made them a fortune, like Méglin's pills, or sedatives with a phenobarbitone base, which were given in small doses or, as was said, 'in divided doses', taken five or six times throughout the day.

A closer examination of the patients showed that the two essential elements in the problem were psychological tension, which led to a physical tension of the body and muscles, and also the concentration and fixation of the patient's mind on a topic of preoccupation, which monopolized the whole field of awareness. The only worthwhile solutions at the time when these first observations were made were to induce a twilight state of drowsiness with large doses of sedatives, which limited the activity of the subject, who had difficulty in working under these conditions; otherwise the suggestion was made to get rid of the preoccupations with leisure pursuits or organized activities, or alternatively voyages, although these were not possible for everybody.

In brief, what was needed to reassure and tranquillize these patients was a double action:

- relax the mind and the body to give free range to a good mood;
- abolish the fixed concentration on an obsessional fear in order to banish anguish and anxiety.

In these two proposals can be found the definition of what a tranquillizer must do; but are these observations not outstandingly trite? People have always striven to achieve this. Well before our grandmothers' herbal tea, Méglin's pills, the bromides and barbiturates, people discovered how to relax mind and body and drive away despondent ideas by drinking alcohol.

Is alcohol the ancestor of the tranquillizers?

Let me make it plain—my aim is not to deliver a panegyric on alcohol, nor to explain why people drink too much. Nevertheless, in this chapter on tranquillizers, I would like to acknowledge alcohol's ancestral role as the precursor in this class of drugs, to explain why humans drink alcohol, all the more so since what is called in chemistry the 'alcohol function' gave birth to the first and one of the best-known modern tranquillizers.

Alcohol is not a food, and it does not increase the capacity for work in healthy people. Its energy content is only shown in increasing deviations in our metabolism, which weigh down our body with adipose tissue. Considered as a drink, and given that it is never drunk at strengths of 90° or 100°, but always diluted in aqueous liquids, it can be said that drinking alcohol is a more or less agreeable way of drinking water.

I am always surprised that puritan moralists, who from one time to another succeeded in getting laws on alcohol restriction passed, have not been held back in their zeal by what they could read in the Bible, where a good number of verses for tens of centuries praise the juice of the vine, this 'plant of quality' that Ecclesiastes recommends drinking, 'providing one behaves in a manner pleasing to God'. When God wishes to punish his people he tells them, 'You will tend your vines, but you will not harvest any because it will be eaten by worms.' Christ drank wine like anybody else, and the Pharisees treated him as *potor vini*, drinker of wine. Of the twenty-four parables contained in the synoptic gospels, four are devoted to the theme of the vine and wine. Wine was highly regarded in antiquity. Greek mythology made the vine the gift of a divinity, surrounded by enthusiastic worship, and wine is also an essential part of the Christian ritual.

Ever since human beings saw the sweet juices fermenting, this drink has been preferred above all others. Why? Perhaps for reasons associated with the physiology of taste—to break up the monotony of consuming water with a drink that tastes more pleasant? It is possible. But our ancestors quickly realized that alcohol not only satisfied thirst, but created a change of mood, eased the sadness of life, and brought an elation that gave fresh vigour. Euphoria, relaxation and oblivion—are these not the qualities we are asking for from tranquillizers? Alcohol has been providing these for a very long time.

Wine and mood

'Oh! Wine! Lift my soul from everyday life, steer it towards another way where it will not be imprisoned in the straight and narrow monotony of my days, where it will not be crushed by sadness and boredom, and see to it that it gives way to gaiety, to the happiness of the moment, and to forgetfulness.' [Hesiod, *Works and Days*]

She loved wine, that Egyptian lady of the Sixth Dynasty who suggested, when offering it to her neighbour at the table:

'Cheer up. See how I love drunkenness, which is so necessary to me. I need eighteen cups of wine.'

Socrates said, 'It seemed right to me that one should drink, for wine comforts the soul, soothes sorrow better than mandrake, and arouses joy just as oil makes the fire burn up.'

Philip II of Macedon learnt to drink very young, but it is said that he became truly alcoholic in the course of his campaigns against the Balkan barbarians, and I think he also must have needed a drink when Demosthenes harangued him and denounced his harmful actions in the *Philippics*.

Should one see in Alexander the Great's drunkenness an alcoholic heredity transmitted through his father? Or did the risks of his inordinate ventures, and of his grandiose conquests, maintain in Philip's son ceaseless tension in respect of the problems to be solved, and the need to drive away fear and reduce indecision? Alexander the Great drank hugely; it is said that his drunken bouts lasted two days and two nights, and that he came to a premature end through drink.

The communal meals of the early Christians involved wine and St Paul tells us about those who got drunk at them. Novatian, one of the Church fathers, tries to explain through mystic anguish the drinking tendency of his flock, who 'young again begin to drink and tip wine into their glasses which are already empty again, and without having eaten, are already drunk.'

Also drinkers were emperors, crowned heads of Europe, Alexander V, Sixtus V, Nicholas V, Leon X. Erasmus, speaking about congregations of monks, tells us, 'What else have they got to relieve their boredom, if it is not to live and drink?'

It was not for the same reasons that the great physician and surgeon Ambroise Paré praised brandy: 'A kind of panacea whose virtues are infinite.' He used it when dressing wounds, but noticed that 'those who, from choice, drink it in moderation find, as well as pleasure in consuming it, a worthy confidence which lets them forget their worries and helps them stay alive.'

Why not end this historical recalling of the effects of alcohol with the praises which Clement of Alexandria awards to wine?

'It makes the mood happier, the judgement clearer, and intercourse with strangers and servants gentler. It is the friend of a countless crowd of unfortunates at the time of their mental misery. In the hours of worry and dejection, it has gladdened their heart. In hours of happiness, it brings it on quicker. In sadness, worry and fear, it restored equilibrium. It has removed the bad mood from their face, given peace to the desperate, the embittered, the anxious, and has let them glimpse for a few hours the rich first light of a new and better day.'

To listen to Clement, is not alcohol the best tranquillizer in the world?

From mead to the honeymoon and psychoanalysis

The alcoholic fermentation of honeyed water produces mead, one of the earliest alcoholic drinks described. In the *Skáldskaparmál*, part of the prose *Edda*, a collection of Icelandic mythological tales, Snorri Sturlason recounts how the dwarfs Fjalarr and Galarr murdered the sage Kvasir, mixed his blood with honey and fermented a potion that passed on to all who drank it sexual energy and the gift of song. Perhaps this is why Scandinavians had a passion for mead. They took this drink to England and it played a major part in ceremonies—particularly nuptial ceremonies, which lasted thirty days, or, more precisely, four weeks and a day, that is to say, a lunar month. The cup of mead was not only an official gift for the husband, but the frequently refilled bowl of mead was perhaps to initiate him in fine songs, devoted to his wife, but also to give him all the qualities needed to fulfil his conjugal duties. It is thought that the expression 'honeymoon', which consecrates the first month after the wedding, can also evoke the stimulating absorption of mead, which lifted the barriers of timidity and reserve which might have inhibited the Scandinavian spouses and their successors.

Before analysing the mechanisms through which alcohol acts as a tranquillizer, let us see what the psychoanalysts who have thoroughly analysed its action have to say about it.

The consumption of alcohol, they say, is a voluntary act whose results are at the same time conscious and unconscious. For the early psychoanalysts, alcohol reduced repressions by its disinhibiting effect. All constraints are relaxed, and the individual temporarily finds a sort of infantile happiness. Some of the repressed tendencies are verbal, but there are also sexual and aggressive impulses.

Alcohol is capable of temporarily relieving anybody suffering from timidity, inferiority feelings or sexual impotence to the degree that, in that individual, it can combat anguish, shame, blame or feelings of insecurity.

Psychopharmacology of alcohol

We must now see if, from the point of view of its mechanism of action, alcohol conforms to the specifications of a tranquillizer, which are essentially:

- to relax the mind and body;
- to scatter lines of thought to dispel anguish and anxiety.

Alcohol is an organic solvent; it is a general poison for cell protoplasm, most noticeably in nerve cells. This action, which depends on the degree of the alcoholic permeation, has several phases.

First, there is a phase of initial excitation, attributable either to direct action on the motor centres, or paresis of the inhibitor centres. In fact the latter mechanism is mainly responsible; alcohol depresses the surface of the brain, which in general controls the underlying structures. At this stage, euphoria develops, with subjective diminution in fatigue.

In the second phase, the depressive action of alcohol takes effect on sensitivity. Pain sensitivity is the first to go, tactile sensitivity lasts longer. There is generally an elimination of unpleasant sensations, in a state where pleasant sensory impressions are still perceived. Progressively, the higher cerebral functions—perceptions, association of ideas, judgement—are affected up to the stage when they are paralysed, if the permeation continues as far as alcoholic coma.

And so two phases of alcoholic intoxication correspond to a tranquilizing effect:

- the initial phase of euphoria, which is not exactly a relaxation, or a loosening up, but which ends with the same result—a good mood;
- the phase of early drunkenness, which dulls perceptions, associations and judgement, and disperses, lessens and drives away anguish and anxiety.

Thus alcohol modifies the links and hierarchies between the base and the surface of the brain where impulses coming from the lower instinctive-affective zones rise to the surface, at the same time as the superior functions are less sensitive to disagreeable perceptions.

If we now think about consciousness, this is what selects and displays our links with the exterior, as well as our perceptions, feelings, states of mind, our pleasure or our anguish, funnelling them in a ruthless manner. If we always had to remain in a wakeful state, we would be driven to complete exhaustion, which would compromise our mental equilibrium. This is when sleep intervenes, coming with regular rhythm to abolish our activity and thoughts, and suppress our links with the outside world. Sleep, in extinguishing our consciousness (to sleep to forget), gives autonomy to other nervous centres, which can thus relax.

Now, what does drunkenness induced by alcohol do? The same thing as sleep; it reduces links with the outside world. However, unlike the drowsiness of sleep, the activity of the exchanges in drunkenness is even greater than in the state of conscious wakefulness. In a manner a good deal more effective than sleep, it can facilitate changes of nerve associations, and modifications of the mind, enabling the dispersal of disagreeable sensations and perceptions with preservation of elementary sensory impressions.

Thus alcohol fulfils its mission as a tranquillizer only in the initial phases, for progression to the terminal phase represents a great risk, which unfortunately can neither be foreseen nor assessed.

The power and danger of drunkenness

Humans have long sought the consoling and tranquillizing properties of alcohol in the bottom of a glass, and found happiness in intoxication. But use can also lead to misuse, especially for alcohol, where tolerance and toxicity can vary considerably from one individual to another. Some can drink heavily for a long time; others quickly find a threshold to their tolerance and cannot stabilize themselves in the euphoric or mild intoxication phase. The absorption of further alcohol then leads to toxic drunkenness in which the lower nerve centres become progressively paralysed. This phase, unlike the euphoric and excitation phases at the beginning, is an essentially depressive phase, which will persist for a long time with the heavy sleep of the drunkard. When the drinker sobers up and awakens, the feelings of anxiety and anguish—from which drinking was an escape—will return, augmented by feelings of blame and shame provoked by the alcohol abuse. What is left for this unhappy, helpless person, full of remorse and anguish, to do? Start to drink again, both to recover the initial euphoria and the exhilarating drunkenness, and also to banish blame and self-accusation. The infernal cycle of alcoholic addiction sets in, transforming the lost soul of today into a human wreck tomorrow. This is why, in spite of its tranquillizing properties, alcohol cannot be medically prescribed.

The glass of rum traditionally offered in France to someone condemned to death on the morning of his execution was justifiable on account of the classical power attributed to alcohol and the absence, in this situation, of the risk of addiction. What would have happened if the condemned person had asked for a double dose of Valium or Tranxene? Only a doctor would have been able to legally prescribe them.

Freedom for alcohol, legal restrictions for the tranquillizers: paradoxically, the dangers and toxicity of one are dismissed in the freedom to drink, whilst the others require medical supervision. This is the essential difference between alcohol and the tranquillizers, the discovery of which we are going to discuss.

The benefits of tranquillizers

Betel and Gajare's problems

The elephants blocked the road, and the three minibuses had to stop to let them pass. They were lugging enormous blocks of teak, towards a nearby sawmill. My travel companions climbed out to take pictures of them, and immediately the elephant drivers' assistants held out their hands to collect rupees. Gajare, our guide, also got down from the vehicle and made up a plug of betel for himself. I have been watching him for two days and find him worried and anxious. On leaving Colombo we stopped at the Negombo market, and he showed us betel-leaf sellers. When I asked him if he chewed betel, he told me with a smile, 'Only when I have problems.'

And for two days, Gajare Desouza chews continuously. Yesterday I counted at least eight plugs, and this is already the fourth this morning— and it is only ten o'clock.

'Gajare, I would like to chew betel. Can you make me up a plug?'

I had wanted to try it since I arrived in Sri Lanka, but had not dared; and the old ladies who sell the leaves and the things to put inside are so dirty that it put me off. With Gajare it would not be the same thing. He buys fresh leaves each morning, of a fine, delicate green, and at the market at Kandy he acquired a supply of about ten areca nuts, some cloves, and some tiny black seeds. Also at the Kandy market, he bought from a fishmonger a white paste with which he filled a very handsome silver box.

Gajare made up a plug for me, not too big and without any clove, tobacco or catechu seeds, which are the seeds of the betel tree. From his bag of leaves, which he kept in a damp towel, he chose a small one, in which he put some pieces of areca nut, then, with a spatula, he took some of the white paste from the silver box, and carefully mixed it with some small pieces of nut. He folded the leaf over the mixture of nut and white paste, and rolled it up as one does with the vine leaves and seasoned rice eaten in Greek or Turkish restaurants. The whole thing was no bigger than a small cork, and of the same shape.

I wanted to know what the white paste was. Gajare showed me his silver box. The paste is slightly gritty, the grains must be felt under the teeth and on the gums; it consists of powdered sea-shells which have been ground up, then calcinated and mixed with water—in other words, lime, which will draw out the oils and active plant alkaloids from the areca nut and the betel leaves. It is indeed a veritable little chemical factory which I am putting between my teeth. I look at Gajare, who is watching me. I have not bitten into the plug yet . . .

'Careful! You must spit first, two or three times.'

'Spit what?'

Gajare puts a plug in his own mouth; a big plug with tobacco, a clove, and a pinch of cooking salt. His cheek is puffed out like a trumpeter. He has not chewed yet either.

'Saliva. You will see, as soon as you have chewed you cannot keep the saliva in.'

Gajare, at the end of his sentence, begins to chew, and I do the same. In a few seconds, a flood of saliva spurts out between my teeth. I stop chewing my plug, which I slip between my cheek and my gum, but nothing will dry up the gush of saliva which now fills my mouth: I have to either spit or swallow.

'Spit! Go on! That's it! Spit first . . .'

I spit on the road a stream of reddish saliva, which splashes up like blood. The handkerchief with which I wipe my lips is stained crimson. My mouth has already refilled with saliva, and I spit again. Gajare is looking at me all the time.

'Spit once more, and after that, swallow.'

He himself has not spat at all, and when I ask him why not, he calmly answers:

'I'm used to it.'

Now, I cautiously swallow half a mouthful and spit out the rest. The taste is tolerable, both lightly astringent and spicy, but a pleasant aromatic and fresh flavour stays in my mouth. Then there is a hot taste again when I bite my plug. Strangely, my salivation has dried up considerably, although I spit out one out of every two mouthfuls. Gajare keeps an eye on me, watching my movements, but he seems to me to be worried all the time. He is pale-skinned with blond hair, a 'burgher': a descendant of mixed Tamil and Portuguese race. With such blond hair I would have bet on Dutch ancestry, but his name is Desouza.

'Gajare, why have you been chewing betel since we were at Kandy?'

He shrugged his shoulders. I pressed him.

'You told me at Negombo that you chew when you have problems. What's wrong?'

He suddenly remembered saying this to me, and now regretted it. I pressed again:

'What's wrong?'

Gajare took me by the arm and pointed out the vehicle at the head of our little convoy to me. In the driver's seat, the driver was sitting with his arms and head folded over the steering wheel.

'You see, that's Badula. He is ill, and this is worrying me very much.'

When we had had breakfast this morning at Galoya, Badula had seemed to me to be in good health.

'It's in his head that he is ill,' Gajare explains. 'His mind is in a whirl.'

I wanted to ask for more details but again my mouth was full of saliva and I went off to go and spit into a ditch. My travel companions got back into the minibuses. I hesitated to hang onto my plug. How would I get on in the bus? Impossible to spit, and all my handkerchiefs would not have been enough. So, swallow all my saliva? I was beginning to develop a liking for the hot taste of my plug, and the perfume which had pervaded my mouth. I decided to keep it. I sat down next to Gajare in the bus which brought up the rear of our procession.

'What's the trouble with Badula?'

Perhaps I am obstinate, but Gajare's worry was preoccupying me. I succeeded in getting the story of what was troubling Gajare and why he had been chewing betel since we were at Kandy.

Badula's anguish

Everything had started at Kandy. We had arrived in the ancient capital of Sri Lanka at the end of the afternoon, and although it was late, Gajare had planned a visit to the tropical garden of Peradeniya. This is one of the two most beautiful botanical gardens in the world; the other is that at Pamplemouse on Maurice Island.

We lingered along the palm grove paths and in the orchid houses, listening to Kalibur, the old guide, spouting his classical lecture on vegetable essences. On getting back to Kandy the front bus, driven by Badula, had pulled up in front of a small Hindu temple, and the two other coaches had stopped; but Gajare leapt to the ground, had some negotiations with Badula, then our procession started off again.

Badula had wanted to perform his devotions to Ganesh, in the Ceruela temple consecrated to chauffeurs and drivers of buses and all other vehicles.

'When you perform your devotions in this temple, at least once a year,' Gajare explained to me, 'you never have an accident. But I know Badula; it would have gone on for almost an hour and we had to get to the Temple of the Tooth before eight o'clock to avoid the crowds.'

Gajare had promised that we would come back to the Ceruela temple on the way out from Kandy the next morning. But we had had to wait for one member of our group who had been unwell during the night and had got up late, and to keep to the timetable Gajare had withdrawn his promise to Badula. We left for Matale without performing the devotions to Ganesh at the Ceruela drivers' temple.

I had noticed the violent dispute between our guide and his drivers as we left Kandy, but as they spoke in Tamil, I had not understood the reasons for the altercation. Of the three drivers in our tour, Badula had been the most angry and the most threatening towards Gajare. The guide's position in charge, responsible for everything on our expedition, had brought him up against the demands of faith and religious superstition. And Badula had threatened to leave the tour.

'If he abandons his job I won't know what to do. I do not have the authority to replace him,' Gajare told me. 'I can drive these minibuses myself all right, but I would be taken to task by all the unions, and even my boss at the agency would disown me.'

What Gajare feared even more was the panic and anxiety of Badula, who was now bound to have an accident. He had caught him the same morning in the process of exorcizing his vehicle with sticks of incense which he had lit and run over the bumpers, tyres, under the bonnet, and inside, over the steering wheel and dashboard. This was why Gajare was chewing betel: to escape from his annoyance and the troubles he believed he had with Badula.

We left the surroundings of the elephants' sawmills and passed along beside a little river which flowed between bamboo hedges when suddenly we came out on to the edge of a plateau: from there we had a view, as far as the eye could see, of thick jungle, from which rose, like an island in this verdant sea, the hill of Sigirya.

Right at the top of this hill the Sinhalese king Kasyapa, who had gone mad, had had a fortress built, reached by a very steep road. We were going to picnic in the castle ruins at the top of the citadel under the benevolent eye of the damsels of Sigirya, guardians of the premises.

In spite of the heat, we climbed the steep path that reached through narrow defiles as far as the first earth platform; but after passing through a gateway across the ramparts it was necessary to follow a path without a parapet, overhanging the void. The view was magnificent, but unsettling and vertiginous, all the more so as an open-work suspension bridge ended the pathway in front of the 'Damsels' Lodge', a kind of open cavern whose walls were embellished with frescos. Heads erect, brown hair smoothed down over wide foreheads crossed by thick eyebrows, the young damsels of the Sigirya frescoes were waiting for us as they must have welcomed King Kasyapa six hundred years ago. The dark eyes and smiling lips wished us welcome, and also offered us the promise of a relaxation which their supple and half-naked bodies indicated in a reverential but provocative way.

We contemplated these gorgeous paintings for a little while, then by a passage which led to the rampart walk we reached the last earth platform. Sheltered from the sun by sections of a high wall that were still standing, we sat down while our guide and drivers handed out food cartons for our lunch.

Suddenly I turned, alerted by a cry, or rather a kind of howling, bursting out behind me. Leaning against a wall of the platform, his head against a barbican, arms and legs outstretched, our driver Badula was screaming with terror. We rushed towards him. He agreed to speak (Gajare translated for us): Badula had suddenly felt that his last moments had arrived. He knew he would never return to the foot of the hill: the fortress of Sigirya would be his tomb. At any rate, nothing could stop him dying. If it was not there, on this platform, it would be on the road, as soon as we had finished our stop.

We tried in vain to calm him down and draw him into the middle of the platform. Tense and on edge, trembling, head and neck stiff, he remained stuck, leaning against the wall. He would not move. By now, not only Gajare but all the members of our group were confronted with a worrying situation. We could not leave Badula in this state, at the top of the Sigirya fortress; and there was no question of forcing him down the perilous footpath and across the suspension bridges, which were the only ways out of the fortress.

I do not know what it was that keep me in good spirits and mobile that day. Perhaps the imposing scenery surrounding us, the combined beauty of the vast green jungle and the dazzling ruins under the tropical sun. Perhaps it was the timeless and magical vision of the damsels of Sigirya. Above all, I think, it was the stimulating effect of my betel plug that gave me the courage and strength to tear down the steep path at top speed, followed by Gajare, to collect the medical kit which goes with me on all my journeys; and, more difficult still, to climb back up the path in the scorching midday heat, cross the bridges and the slope, and reach the citadel platform in record time.

Badula was still in the same state of shaking and anguish as when we had left him. The two other drivers were beside him, almost as worried as he was. I approached him to speak to him in an English which he understood. Badula was not hallucinating or delirious. He was dragged into a huge whirlpool of scruples and moral dilemmas. His sworn religion, which must be kept to, did not accept the involuntary betrayal of not having observed the pilgrimage to Ganesh of the Ceruela. He was crucified by remorse that he could not dispel. His spirit and his mind were strained, tense at the thought of his disobedience to his faith, and his attention was fixed on the punishment that the gods would inflict upon him there, in this wild and terrible setting of the ancient ruined fortress.

I negotiated with Badula, with my medicine box under my arm; I do not remember now what I told him, but with his friends the drivers, and with Gajare the guide, we all recalled everything, from the gods of all countries, his family and his children, the power of my pills, the journey that must be completed, the troubles he was going to make for himself with the company who hired the buses, and finally the untenable state of his standpoint there, at the top of these ruins where he could not remain.

Badula was willing to swallow the three tablets which I gave him, with water from our gourds, and I also made him eat half an orange. We waited patiently for the effect of my drugs to make themselves felt, while our travel companions went down to the foot of the hill. At the end of three-quarters of an hour, Badula was calm; he asked for more to drink, his limbs were no longer tensed on the stone table where he had been seated, and his head was moving every now and then from side to side. He lifted his hand and spoke in Tamil to Gajare, calmly enough; long sentences, punctuated with gestures in which he indicated me. Gajare answered him equally calmly and seemed to be agreeing with what Badula was saying. At one point the guide put his hand on Badula's shoulder, giving him a friendly tap. Everything seemed to be going for the better.

'He says that your medicine is as powerful as the water of the Yan Oya spring, which gives peace. He thinks that Ganesh will pardon him, but he must go back to the temple of Ceruela before the end of the year, and I have promised him that I will take him as a driver on the next tour which is going to Peradeniya. He is quite willing to go down now.'

I was pleased that Badula had decided so quickly, for I had rather pushed the dose of diazepam (Valium) that I had given him, and it was better for him to go down on his own, or supported, rather than be carried down the dangerous path. When we got back to his minibus he was staggering a bit, but nevertheless wanted to drive; we dissuaded him, and Gajare took his place at the wheel. After a short time, he dozed off in the vehicle. On arriving at Polonnaruwa, which marked the end of the stage, Badula had woken up. For the days which followed, he remained very calm. Each evening I gave him a Valium tablet, and he drove his vehicle again the next morning.

At the time of our visit to the Galoya reserve, I was relaxing one evening on the rest-house veranda to watch the sunset over the lake. Gajare, followed by his three drivers, came over to me.

'We'd like to know what you gave Badula on the hill at Sigirya.'

I asked why they wanted to know.

'Because these tablets get rid of fear.'

Badula's fear of having displeased the god Ganesh, Gajare's fear because of Badula's behaviour, and the other drivers' fear of suffering the same fate as Badula. These men of Sri Lanka were affected by fear of fear itself, producing the same anguish in their wild, beautiful island that people experience in the noisy cities of Europe.

The four men were standing in front of me, back by the setting sun, their silhouettes dark against the waters of Galoya, which stretched from beyond the terrace to the islands of black rocks where white eagles slept in dead trees. How, on this peaceful evening, could anyone think about tomorrow's distress? These men were like so many others: frightened of fear, and hoping for happiness through equanimity, tranquillity and peace.

I said I would tell them the name of my medication when we got back to Colombo.

This exotic tale, marked by the superstition of a Tamil faithful to the god Ganesh, but where betel-chewing and Valium-taking also come in, deserves no other conclusion perhaps than these two questions which I should be asked, and which I also ask myself. Why had I wanted to chew betel? And why did I have Valium in my medicine box?

If curiosity and the desire to understand better than by watching or questioning others had pushed me to experiment myself with betel, which millions of individuals in the world chew every day, to no great harm, why, in putting together my medicine box for travelling, had I included a tranquillizer?

Panaceas?

Evolution and progress, development and refinement of science and technology, have upset routine. It is the duty of fashion, in so far as it is only the taste of the day, to bring our knowledge up to date and to plan our way of living, and even of dying. Fifty years ago, when asked to name the three medicines they would like to have available on a desert island, doctors chose aspirin, tincture of iodine, and morphine. Aspirin already had its reputation as a universal medication. Tincture of iodine was the ideal surgical antiseptic, and morphine helped with dying. Times have changed. I would retain aspirin in this list, but I would exchange tincture of iodine for a polyvalent antibiotic for use internally and possibly externally, and I would replace morphine with diazepam or another tranquillizer of the same strength.

With aspirin, an antibiotic and diazepam, I would be able to look after a hundred times as many patients on my desert island than with the former triad, more effectively, and with less risk.

Certainly a large part of this progress is due to the antibiotic, but the diazepam offers many therapeutic possibilities in addition to its tranquilizing effect. For apart from psychological indications, the use of tranquilizers is so frequent and varied that they are amongst the most commonly prescribed drugs in medicine today. All psychosomatic disturbances may benefit from tranquillizing drugs, whether they be digestive, cardiovascular, dermatological or other troubles. For gastric or intestinal spasms, nervous coughs, palpitations, skin irritations, some allergies, and many other pathological conditions are often provoked or accentuated by anxiety, anguish or groundless fears. *The effect of tranquillizers on symptoms is unquestionable*; and if they do not represent a fundamental treatment, they are as essential in some cases as the drugs that treat the underlying problem. It could even be said that in every pathological disorder, if a bed is needed for the sick body to lie on, the tranquillizer is the divan on which the tormented mind finds peace.

The agitation of the anxious, their sleep difficulties, the spasms of the lump in the throat, or the hand with cramp, and even unstable behaviour and nocturnal terrors in children are thus all cared for. One must beware, however, of other organic or psychiatric disorders that may be masked by these symptoms, and whose underlying cause must be identified and treated.

Let us see how the first tranquillizers were found.

Origin of the first tranquillizers

Because it is not without benefit to go back to origins, even if only to extol the inventor, and because everyone thinks that the first tranquillizer came from America, we are going to France to start our pilgrimage to the source.

It is 1910, and the Poulenc brothers have just marketed a new drug under the name Antodyne. This product was synthesized by a team of chemists directed by Ernest Fourneau, whose extraordinary talents have been sadly overlooked; for the discovery of antisyphilitics, antimalarials, sulphonamides, and many other products are due to him. Fourneau, who was one of the first pharmacological chemists, and who trained such pupils as Daniel Bovet and Bernard Halpern, became interested in phenoxypropanediol, which was the active ingredient of Antodyne.

Now, as the etymology of the trade name indicates, Antodyne was a calming agent, and amongst the indications mentioned in the prospectus was included 'insomnia due to nervous excitation'.

Antodyne can be considered as the ancestor of the tranquillizers, for the first product that the American Frank Berger spoke of as an 'anti-anxiety tranquillizer' was methylphenoxypropanediol, still known under the name of mephenesin. Only a small methyl group distinguishes Fourneau's Antodyne from Mallinson, Berger and Schlan's mephenesin. It was between the years 1946 and 1949 that first the antispasmodic and relaxing properties of mephenesin, then its tranquillizing properties, were discovered.

I have already explained how a mental relaxation and a muscular relaxing action can be linked, and how one can trigger off the other. I have also related how, using curare, physical and psychological relaxation can be obtained through infracurarization. Going back to the definition of a tranquillizer, which is a product that 'relaxes the mind and the body', every muscle relaxant must have a tranquillizing action.

To relax the muscle, the excitatory nerve must be inhibited or, better, paralysed. Now there are two places where nerve impulses may be suppressed: at the level where the nerve enters the muscle (which is where curare works), or at the level where the nerve leaves the spinal cord—and that is where the relaxing tranquillizers like mephenesin act.

The tranquillizing relaxants

It is known that if the spinal cord is divided, as can happen in fractures of the vertebral column, paralysis of all the nerves and all the muscles below the fracture level results. Now, there are chemical products that, without destroying the spinal cord, can poison it for a short while, and reduce its ability to transmit spontaneous and reflex nerve and muscle activity. These drugs are called 'medullary depressants'. When the cord is depressed, so too is the nerve, and the muscle relaxes. So the medullary depressants are also muscular relaxants, and consequently psychological relaxants as well, and thus they are tranquillizers.

Berger and Bradley analysed the action of mephenesin (Décontractyl) as a medullary depressant in 1946. Mallinson recommended the drug as a muscle relaxant in 1947, and in 1948 Berger, with Schwartz, Schlan and Unna, demonstrated its psychological relaxant action. The authors showed that mephenesin could soothe anxiety without affecting consciousness or causing sleep.

If one looks at the dates, it can be appreciated that 'tranquillizing' activity became known in 1948, well before 'neuroleptic' activity, which only dates from 1952. At the time, the word 'sedative' covered tranquillizing effect, and at any rate the 'tranquillizers' of 1948 were no more effective in the psychoses than those discovered in 1952 and 1958.

Mephenesin, which is a derivative of propanediol, is—as its termination in 'ol' indicates—an alcohol (here we find our ancestor of the tranquillizers), and this alcohol has the drawback of being quickly oxidized and destroyed in the body, limiting its activity. An attempt was made to strengthen it by combining phenobarbitone with mephenesin-based drugs (Décontractyl–Phénobarbital) but Berger had the idea of intervening directly on the molecule, into which he introduced an acid derived from urea: carbamic acid. He made a carbamate of mephenesin, but this product's duration of action was no better than that of mephenesin. Then Berger found that by using a different alcohol (methylpropyl-propanediol) and two molecules of carbamic acid, he obtained a stable and powerful chemical compound. He had discovered meprobamate, also called Equanil, Miltown and procalmadiol.

Few people connected meprobamate with a very old chemical compound, urethane, used as a hypnotic; however, urethane is the carbamate of ethyl alcohol (the alcohol one drinks), and meprobamate is the dicarbamate of methylpropylpropanediol (not an alcohol for drinking). There we find our tranquillizing alcohol effect.

However that may be, meprobamate spread throughout the world, and was widely adopted because of its calming, sedative and anxiolytic properties. Discovered in 1952, at the same time as chlorpromazine, meprobamate remained the only valid tranquillizer until the discovery of chlordiazepoxide (Librium) and diazepam (Valium) in 1958.

Here it is necessary to make a clarification that is as useful for the general public as it is for doctors less acquainted with the use of psychotropic drugs.

The discovery of meprobamate and the tranquillizers, their considerable commercial development and their use in therapeutics, has drawn an aura of mystery and a worldwide celebrity around them, and yet, from the scientific, medical and humanitarian point of view, there is no possible comparison between this discovery and that of the neuroleptics such as chlorpromazine. Even with the whole range of current tranquillizers, it would not have been possible to treat and cure psychotic patients, and the therapeutic revolution in the asylums and psychiatric hospitals would not have happened.

On the one hand, with the neuroleptics, the inmates of the asylums have been truly set free. On the other hand, with the tranquillizers, our modern civilization has been provided with 'comfort drugs' that help it stand up better to the noise and frenzy it makes for itself. This is why I think it is wrong to call both categories of drugs 'tranquillizers', even if those that act on psychoses are qualified as 'major', and 'minor' is applied to the psychological comfort drugs, for confusion arises if the two qualifications of 'major' and 'minor' are not included. This is how it could be said that alcohol was not a tranquillizer because it did not work in psychoses, whilst meprobamate, which does not work for mental illness either, is one. To sum up, classification into neuroleptics—drugs for psychoses—and tranquillizers—drugs for psychological comfort—is greatly preferable and should be accepted and brought into general use throughout the world, as it already is in Europe.

Discovery of the anxiolytic tranquillizers

Meprobamate relaxes the mind and the body. Is this through its muscle relaxant properties? This is possible. I am inclined to favour a euphoric action as well, comparable to that provided by alcohol, certainly with fewer disadvantages than the latter when one has drunk too much, for there is no hangover or reactionary depression. There are other grounds for supporting my meprobamate–alcohol comparison. In delirium tremens caused by acute alcohol poisoning, meprobamate perfused intravenously acts outstandingly well on the attack of mental confusion. It is known that at one time 25% intravenous alcohol (Curéthy) was given to these patients, and they tolerated this without harm.

This relaxing action of meprobamate, helpful for many anxious and worried people, has sometimes been found inadequate when a fear or obsessive worry takes over the whole of the mind. It is in these cases that in place of the relaxing tranquillizers, anxiolytic tranquillizers can be used, like diazepam (Valium), clorazepate (Tranxène) or medazepam

(Nobrium), which are all derived from chlordiazepoxide (Librium), discovered by the researchers at the Hoffmann–La Roche company.

In 1955 the chemist Leo Sternbach made forty quinazoline derivatives, all of which were inactive in the laboratory. Somewhat disappointed, he processed one of the last products using a chemical compound slightly different from those he had used for the preceding forty molecules. However, this last product, unlike the others, was not studied. It was not until a year later that Lowell Randall, a pharmacologist at Hoffmann–La Roche, undertook the study of this compound, RO-5-0690. On 27 July 1957 Dr Randall wrote in a report, 'The product has hypnotic, sedative, and strychnine antagonist properties in the mouse identical to that of meprobamate.' Unlike the forty other preceding products, not only was RO-5-0690 active, it also had a different chemical structure; it was a completely new compound, originating from an unsuspected molecular rearrangement.

The first clinical trials of this product began at the start of 1958, and came to nothing. But Dr Hines, director of biological research at the Hoffmann–La Roche laboratories, asked for new studies to be undertaken because he had noticed that RO-5-0690 had a quite specific and original action on animals—that of facilitating their training. He even had a film made showing ferocious animals, tigers, panthers, pumas and particularly aggressive monkeys, which became quite calm with RO-5-0690; they could then be approached without danger, as if they had been trained.

New studies in psychiatric clinics and on voluntary patients were undertaken by Irving Cohen, James Sussex and Titus Harris. On 12 March 1960, in the *Journal of the American Medical Association*, Harris published the first report describing the tranquillizing action of chlordiazepoxide, which was marketed the same year under the name of Librium. A few years later diazepam, a more powerful related compound, was in turn suggested for therapeutics.

These tranquillizers, the benzodiazepines, have the property of detaching the patient's attention from matters of emotional fixation, diverting and dispelling sorrow and distress, by eliminating haunting fears that have become obsessions, giving rise to anguish and anxiety. Their mode of action has long remained a mystery, but recently the neuromediator system may have been found through which they intervene in cerebral metabolism. This involves gamma-aminobutyric acid (GABA), whose role was already known in other phenomena regulating vigilance. However that may be, the benzodiazepines have become, through the widespread nature of their use and the ever-increasing call for their prescription, everyday objects of consumption by people allergic to modern life.

What is a tranquillizer worth?

It is futile to argue too much about the facts of this world when they are only the scenery of life's tragicomedy that we act out in the costumes and make-up we have chosen. The tranquillizers help us to play our part when we have stage-fright at the thought of appearing before our public, and, above all, before ourselves. If general practitioners or psychiatrists prescribe them, they must do so advisedly to treat the symptoms for which they have been shown to be effective. Their use must stop as soon as the performance is over. To go on to prescribing tranquillizers as soon as a patient snivels or groans would be to take a step in the direction of bringing these drugs into general use for most illnesses of any kind. Tranquillizers should not be prescribed automatically for people who show vague symptoms or problems associated with a tiresome psychological situation. One must listen, question, analyse, and try to resolve the conflict, only giving tranquillizers if this is necessary, and leaving them off once cure has occurred; this is an absolute rule. In contrast to the neuroleptics, which must be given in regular doses to psychiatric patients for years, the tranquillizers, if prescribed or used without stopping, can lead to addiction problems. Withdrawal problems have certainly been reported in some tranquillizer addicts.

It must also be appreciated that tranquillizers are potentiated by alcohol and that reflexes and vigilance are then reduced, which may lead to the risk of accidents for motorists. In too heavy doses, tranquillizers given during the day may diminish intellectual activity and professional work output. Finally, administered for overlong periods, tranquillizers diminish sexual activity; although they have been used with good results, in particular cases, to treat impotence.

Tranquillizers have been in use for many years, and it appears that, judiciously prescribed, they are not dangerous drugs; but they must be taken under medical supervision. Because their use is so widespread, they have been styled 'psychological aspirins'. This is an oversimplification, but it should be remembered that even aspirin has a certain toxicity, which thoughtless use aggravates.

If I had to judge tranquillizers on their greatest virtue I would look for it away from the controversies they raise, in the calmness and peace they bring to minds oppressed by fear. For their essential merit is to disperse the restlessness and widespread fear that give rise to anguish, making them disappear, or at least hiding them under a mask of placid serenity.

6
The future of psychiatric medicine

Realities and Utopias

The successive discoveries of the neuroleptics, the antidepressants, and finally the tranquillizers, made it possible not only to understand certain aspects of cerebral function better, but also to give general practitioners and psychiatrists drugs that were totally lacking until then. These discoveries have rightly been considered to have completely changed the whole concept and treatment of mental illness. Statistics show globally that there are fewer patients in asylums, that many patients are effectively treated at home, and that others can even work and 'live with their psychoses' while waiting to be cured. This has been called 'made-to-measure treatment', guaranteeing freedom to patients who formerly would never have known it.

The reunion of psychiatry and medicine

This progress in mental health was accompanied by something that I consider even more important, and which I had awaited with impatience since my first encounter with mental illness: the reunion of psychiatry and medicine.

Thanks to psychopharmacology, psychiatry has resumed its place beside the other great medical specialities through the discovery of specific drugs able to satisfy the doctor's therapeutic vocation. This reintegration of mental disturbance as an 'illness' within the framework of medicine was not easily accomplished. From antiquity until the late Middle Ages, mental illness had steered a delicate course between organic conceptions and witch-hunts. From medieval times until the end of the sixteenth century, the gallows and the stake were always ready for those who followed the path of 'twisted reason'. Alone among the doctors of his time, Paracelsus believed that mental illness 'developed in the body, out of disorders of the internal substances which make up the body'. This arrogant alchemist, who declared that 'the hairs on the back of his neck knew more about it than all the authors put together and that the buckles of his shoes contained more wisdom than Avicenna or Galen', said that 'all physical or mental illness could be cured with a specific medicine'.

Unfortunately, through lack of means and appropriate effective treatment, mentally ill patients were condemned to gallows or prison for more than two centuries.

The burning pyre was followed by dungeons and chains to keep those who frightened others, and could not and should not live with others, out of sight. Locked up in cells like criminals, they were left to rot in their excrement. Violent patients were imprisoned in narrow cages or tied up in straitjackets. The rest were chained to the walls or to their beds. Beatings were common, justified on doubtful grounds and given by keepers of low intelligence, or sadists, who could not find any other work. Reil wrote of this period, 'The cries of rage, day and night, of the violent patients, and the clanking of chains made what little reason remained in new arrivals disappear.'

Three reasons justified these atrocities:

- ignorance about the nature of mental illness;
- the fear that it inspired;
- the belief, indeed the certainty, that it was incurable.

It is therefore no surprise that, when Pinel became director of the Bicêtre hospital in 1793, his contemporaries took him to be mad too, because he freed the patients from their chains, gave them air and suitable food, and treated them with kindness.

In spite of Pinel and his successors, the absence of therapeutic results in psychiatry in the nineteenth century was to distance mental pathology more and more from medicine, and to put it in the hands of the asylum doctors who were more nosy psychologists than therapeutic doctors.

The beginning of the twentieth century brought little change. The progress and prestige of neurology with Jean-Martin Charcot and Jules Déjerine, and of psychology with Pierre Janet and Edouard Claparède, did not lead to any effective treatment for mental illness. As for Freud's psychoanalysis, which succeeded in explaining human behaviour in its widest sense in psychological terms, did it have the characteristics of a medical science? There is no agreement over this yet. At any rate, the method it used had nothing to do with any classical medical therapy. And so medicine became 'amputated from psychiatry'—that is to say from the psychiatrists and from the patient, and, in spite of their success, it was certainly not the shock treatments, with their frightening spectacle and mysterious mechanism, that could have brought them together.

This is why, I repeat, the discovery of the neuroleptics in 1952 was a fundamental step in medical research and therapeutics, once more bringing together mental medicine and medicine of the body, through the discovery of drugs active in the psychoses:

- by pacifying mentally disturbed patients, their fears were eliminated;
- in making the patients better, the curability of the psychoses was proved;
- by analysing the action of the neuroleptics and the psychotropic drugs, the causes of mental illness began to be fathomed.

Where does this immense progress now lead us? What can we hope for from these discoveries?

Balance, boredom, and anguish

It was chance perhaps—but chance singularly supported by the painstaking and scientific spirit of enquiring and learned scientists—that made the more or less fortuitous discovery of the first mind drugs possible. The manufacture of their analogues, and of new products, has proceeded from more cleverly constructed hypotheses and delicate biochemical studies, and meticulous observations of their actions. The progress of cerebral chemistry and the neurochemistry of the mediators and transmitters is sure to make it possible to develop increasingly specific drugs, and perhaps substances affecting memory, attention, association mechanisms, the active and resting states of the nerve cell, and its ageing and metabolism as well. It is known that, in another field, the hallucinogens, the 'mind poisons', have already shown their powerful psychological action. Conversely, supporting or psychological comfort drugs can be imagined, facilitating our intellectual mechanisms and helping our mental activity.

Some people, naïvely trusting in a science that seems all-powerful to them because they have no experience of it, think that everything can, or will be, possible. They are beginning to dream . . . like Aldous Huxley, filled with enthusiasm after his mescaline experiments, who called for 'a new drug which will soothe and console our suffering race, without giving rise to social consequences as undesirable as alcohol or the barbiturates, and be less injurious to the heart and lungs as the tar and nicotine in cigarettes . . .' or, closer to our time, the writer Arthur Koestler, who allowed himself to be convinced by certain purely theoretical studies* that minds could be influenced by chemical means.

It is no longer a case of an artificial paradise, nor the 'soma' of the brave new world, nor the happiness drug, but the 'equilibrium pill'. For Koestler, this pill, he tells us in his book *Janus*,

'will provide us with dynamic equilibrium and bring together reason and faith and restore the hierarchical order, by reconciling emotion and reason in normal people, and by strengthening critical facul-

---

* In particular, those of Hyden on the action of tricyanoaminopropene.

ties, and especially by calming the militant, murderous and suicidal enthusiasm which fills the history books just as much as the daily newspapers.'

He adds,

'Certainly, I would rather put my hope in persuasion ... Unfortunately we are a race of "mental patients", deaf to persuasion. This will only be provided by "altering" human nature, and it will be a pill which will do this. An immunizing pill which will confer mental stability.'

And, further, he adds,

'So salvation will be synthesized in the pharmaceutical laboratories. It will no longer be the old alchemist's dream of discovering the elixir of life, but even better than eternal life we will have a pill which transforms homo maniacus into homo sapiens.'

To impose this pill, Koestler will call upon publicity, official encouragement, fashion, well-informed interest, to a referendum, and one could add the product to the drinking water.'

    I will not criticize the author for having switched from a novel into a political essay, and from philosophy to ingenuous fiction; perhaps it is, with age, a logical slip for some. I will also leave to others the task of saying whether this immunizing pill, this 'mental stabilizer', is a materialistic idea or a scientific novelty, for both these possibilities could be overturned by either a detailed critique or become quickly outdated by scientific breakthroughs. But I think that there is no kind of persuasion—or indeed any means of coercion—even subtly with a pill (which if done in the name of liberty would, of course, be a contradiction in terms) that will ever stop us from refusing the prospect of infinite boredom that the promise of mental stability and controlled and regulated emotions would offer us. Human beings, I believe, will always prefer swaying between dreams and reality, unbridled imagination and reason, and freedom to bring forth in their head Don Quixote and Sancho Panza at the same time, to an equilibrium pill. For the hallucinated hidalgo and the realistic horseman have always been complementary in our heads. They must travel along there side by side, between good sense and delirium, between the reality of our external world and the utopia of the imagination. If Rosinante overtakes Sancho's donkey it is perhaps the drama of madness; but if the bourgeois Panza outdistances the knight, it is no more than the boredom of the deserted Castilian behind the donkey's rump.

    People in the future will continue to risk their necks on carefully calculated projects or on throws of the dice. Following their luck, it is often difficult for them to choose between comic opera and tragedy. However, there are also those whose horizon is suddenly covered in mists, who are seized with anguish and the anger of the gods; those who have thrown in their hand in great fear, those whose sad fate it is impossible not to be moved by. Better than happiness pills to treat these poor souls, the road must be found that leads to the hiding place where the world's anguish lurks, sly, and recklessly wicked.

Where is the world's anguish hiding?

The gentlemen of Varenna

Since morning, the inhabitants of Varenna had seen strangers arriving in their village. They were peaceful men, discreet, soberly dressed in well-cut suits. Their luggage was mostly restricted to one case, but they all carried in their hands a briefcase or a gusseted leather bag from which they were never separated.

Many had landed at Milan airport and had taken the train, but some who had come through Switzerland had come by car from St Moritz or from Lugano. Apart from the Italians, almost all had had to work out the location of Varenna, a small village on the east bank of Lake Como, facing Bellagio.

I arrived at Varenna in the evening by the last train from Milan. Through narrow streets, almost deserted and poorly lit, I reached a hotel near the little port. My bedroom was very hot, and the coolness of the evening had not yet set in. After depositing my baggage, I went down to the terrace to find out from my colleagues—I almost said my accomplices—about the programme for the next day's meeting. I learnt that those in charge had, with great care, established a strict protocol. Each member present had to take responsibility for what he said, set the facts out clearly, and suggest logical conclusions that could be verified by everybody.

I had listened to Seymour Kety and Joel Elkes while drinking a glass of iced grappa, in which grains of coffee were floating which I crunched when one slipped through my lips. I ventured:

'If the observed facts and the results obtained lead to a hypothesis not yet verified, the conclusion could be difficult to draw.'

'All new facts, truly original and clearly established, are interesting and deserve being passed on,' said a tall, blond man who had not spoken up till then.

I had never seen him at our meetings. He was introduced to me as Dr Bernard Polis from Philadelphia.

On the way back to my room I asked an American colleague who this Dr Polis was.

'Since this morning, impossible to find out. He was invited directly, as an observer, at his own request, by the organizers,' he answered.

Our meetings were pretty exclusive, so this Dr Polis must have been strongly recommended.

The heat was still considerable in my room, and I did not get off to sleep until late in the night, after I had checked once more that I could, without fear of being criticized, give an account of what I had found.

From Lake Como to the world's anguish

The meeting was to take place in one of the rooms at the Monastero Villa, built in a park whose terraced gardens went down to the lake.

The inaugural session was opened by the general secretary, Jordi Folch-Pi, from Boston; he recalled the object of our gatherings and the specific nature of our discussions, which sought to explain higher nerve functions in chemical terms.

I listened to the speaker without close attention, for I was still reflecting on the results I was going to present. Through one of the windows in the room a view stretched out to Lake Como, whose blue waters, that June morning in 1960, could be made out between the cypresses and oleanders which bordered its shores. I could not stop thinking about whoever it was who had chosen this venue, which was paradoxically so auspicious for our discussions; for in the gardens, in this countryside of peace and tranquillity, by one of the most beautiful Italian lakes, we were going to talk about the world's anguish.

Who had suggested this theme? I no longer remember, but I recall that everyone had been in agreement. Some because they liked dreaming, others because they hoped perhaps to solve insoluble problems. At any rate, it was in free discussions, between the theory sessions, in the Monastero gardens, that this question was going to be tackled.

'Anguish,' said somebody, 'was born for the population of the whole world on 6 August 1945, with the Hiroshima bomb.' Another answered that prehistoric man, long before Hiroshima, had felt anguish on seeing his face reflected in the sea water when he quenched his thirst. The conversation being led by a logician, the true distinction was drawn from the psychological aspect of the question, and of course Freud was mentioned.

Freud had begun by explaining that anguish resulted from frustration of an instinctive search for sexual pleasures, but he soon renounced this definition. In his book *Inhibition, Symptoms and Anxiety* (1926) he defined anguish as an alarm signal at the approach of danger, which mobilizes the defences of the 'self', that is to say, the personality. When the danger comes from an external cause, there is simply fear, but when the danger comes from the threat of the sudden eruption of internal feelings suppressed in the subconscious, this reaction against internal danger is anguish.

This definition and explanation of anguish according to Freud opened the debate, and served to launch a more organic approach to the ques-

tion. It was known that all fear and psychological assaults create disturbances that have repercussions on bodily organs, giving rise to illnesses.
This relation and interdependence between the psychological and the
physical is expressed by detectable organic lesions, but the established
lesion was at a much too advanced stage; what one wanted to catch was
the premonitory phase, before organic disease.

It was first necessary to explain, in detail, what happened in the
human, and see how this could be expressed in the animal, in order to
be able to tackle the chemical—and indeed therapeutic—problems more
easily in the former. For my own part, I had carried out some experiments
about which I was going to talk for the first time at Varenna. But to explain
things better, I am going to call on frames of a film that won the *Palme
d'or* at the Cannes film festival in 1980.

My American uncle's rats

In the film *My American Uncle*, directed by Alain Resnais based on an
idea of Dr Henri Laborit, you see a couple subjected to psychological
trauma, strokes of ill fate, and brutal changes in their way of life, and
reacting to these damaging and anguishing situations with more or less
severe organic, or, as they are called, somatic ailments. One of these
characters had a heart attack and the other a stomach ulcer, set beside
bouts of depression and even suicide attempts. It is a clear demonstration of the repercussion of psychological trauma, anguish, and the reaction to stress and aggression with well-defined organic diseases.

I watched an interview with Laborit on the Croisette at Cannes during
the film festival. His face, which I had known for so long, still reflected the
enthusiasm that inspired the discoverer of the remarkable properties of
chlorpromazine.

He spoke once more about the functions of the brain, which he knew
so well, but also about a certain 'enough is enough' that too often would
be the scene in our lives. He held forth with the conviction that had been
typical of him for thirty years, but in a slightly weary way that surprised
me when he said he had been happy to 'associate his marginality with a
work of art created by Alain Resnais'.

If, instead of listening to him on my small screen, I had been close to
him, I should have told him that his marginality had always given value
and even charm to his scientific work, and when he wearily sighed,
'Tomorrow I shall no longer be there,' I would not have had much of an
answer for this banality we all share.

A few days after this interview, on the occasion of a lunch with Simone
Laborit and Pierre Huguenard, I confided in them that I was going to tell,
in this book, another story about rats, which would perhaps be an answer
to Resnais's film, as I had tried to reply to the 'conspirators of Varenna'.

From the Varenna conspiracy to the hypothalamus

It really was a conspiracy against anguish that the neurochemistry scientists of Varenna were taking part in. It was encircled and pursued, and efforts were made to cut it down. The neuroleptic drugs and antidepressants had slightly lifted the veil that lay over mental illness and melancholia, but the tranquillizers that millions of people took every day to dispel their fears and worries did nothing to help find out where anguish was hiding. The enemy had to be destroyed in a blind combat where the target was not clearly identified. The stomach ulcer, the heart attack and the eruption of eczema were signs of the damage wreaked by anguish, but what we needed to know was from where the weapons had been launched, where the command post was, and where the orders had come from. Where was anguish hiding?

Anguish is first perceived as a psychological phenomenon by the superior and outer part of our brain, by what is called the cerebral cortex. This part of our brain, which essentially distinguishes us from animals, has developed over the course of half a million years of evolution, at a fantastic speed by comparison with all other living things. This higher brain, the cerebral neocortex, is disproportionately large in comparison with the other parts of our brain, in particular the lower brain, also called the limbic brain.

In the upper part, the largest and most recent area of the neocortex, our superior mental functions are seated. In the lower, more primitive (if it can be called that) part is seated our basic affective life, our feelings of hunger, thirst, sexual desire, and our reactions of fight or flight.

So, two brains can be distinguished: the thinking cortical brain and the limbic affective brain; and in the limbic brain, there are three parts that we are going to discuss: the thalamus, where all the sensory pathways are concentrated on their way up to the cortical brain to transmit affective emotions that have arisen in the underlying limbic brain; the *hypothalamus*; and below the hypothalamus, a gland essential for the functioning of our body—a gland that sends orders to all the other glands—the *hypophysis*.

Remember carefully the name of the hypothalamus, this area huddled up between the marshalling yard of the thalamus and the Ali Baba's cave of the hypophysis. It is in the hypothalamus that everything happens. It is from within the hypothalamus that several scientists, including Roger Guillemin, the Frenchman who became a naturalized American, drew their Nobel prizes.

The hypothalamus is where our impulses, good or bad, and our instincts are elaborated, and it is there also where shocks, traumas, countermands and aggressions are perceived; and the impulses or reactions in the hypothalamus will simultaneously pass upwards to the cerebral cortex to be 'intelligently interpreted', and give us pleasure or fright, and pass downwards to the hypophysis to give us hunger or thirst, or elevate our blood pressure, or even ulcerate our stomachs if this is what anguish commands.

For all this we only had indirect proof, because it had been possible to touch, injure or destroy this hypothalamus with Delgado's or Old's needles in order to alter the behaviour of animals. And then, once more, one day ... a way was found to reveal hypothalamic activity under the microscope.

Like a developer on a photographic plate, thanks to a special staining technique discovered by the scientist Gomori, violet-coloured granules were successfully revealed in the hypothalamus; secretions that seemed to move as if under the influence of a current towards the hypophysis. Proof had been found for the secretory activity of the hypothalamus, which gave its orders through the intermediary of these neurosecretions to the hypophysis.

It was not easy to stain the hypothalamus with Gomori's stain. I managed this thanks to the skill of Paul Guiraud, the first to use promethazine in mental illness. He was an exceptional histologist, well versed in all the microscopic staining techniques. He kindly agreed to pass on all the secrets of his methods to my collaborator and friend, Roger Roudier, who was director of the histochemical section of my institute. We then succeeded in establishing precisely the appearance, flow and emptying of Gomori's secretion granules from the hypothalamus into the hypophysis.

What was most interesting, and what represented the most original phenomenon we discovered, was that the extent of these secretions and their presence in the hypothalamus depended upon the conditions of peace or anguish affecting the animals concerned. If the animals were happy, calm and peaceful, there were many Gomori secretory granules in the hypothalamus. If the animals were subjected to stress, aggression, or imminent or prolonged danger, the secretory granules disappeared from the hypothalamus. As if carried by a current, they swept into the hypophysis, where their sudden emergence induced convulsions, hypertension, shock, stomach ulcers, and all the other manifestations of repeated emotional shocks, which Alain Resnais was to illustrate twenty years later in his film, inspired by Laborit.

Thus I had succeeded in identifying the departure point of aggression reactions, the command post where anguish, acting upon the hypothalamus, floods the hypophysis with its secretions. To demonstrate this discovery in a more precise manner, I repeated the experiments using electric shocks in the rat, in particular by bringing about constraint gastric ulcers in the same animal following Dr Bonfils's technique.

If a rat is imprisoned in a cylindrical cage of wire mesh, in which the animal cannot move, either backwards or forwards, and is thus constrained to keep still, at the end of a few hours it develops stomach ulcers as a consequence of the anguish provoked by this constraint. Now, in such rats, no Gomori secretion granules were found in the hypothalamus; in contrast, the hypophysis was filled with them, establishing as a result a reaction that, through the intermediary of suprarenal secretions, provoked the rat's ulcers.

I also showed that electric shock in rats caused the Gomori secretions in the hypothalamus to disappear. Likewise, when certain fish such as guppies or minnows are put into swirling water or water containing slightly irritant substances, they react by changing their colour, by dilating their chromatophores—cells in the interstices of the scales that make coloured pigments appear or disappear.

Now, it is known that constriction or dilatation of the chromatophores in fish is under the influence of the hypophysis, itself regulated by the hypothalamus. So, everything that was a reaction to emotional shock, caused by anguish, seemed indeed to come from this part of the inferior brain, from the limbic brain, from this hypothalamic region.

I also performed some counterchecks, protecting the animals with neuroleptics and tranquillizers. Thus, with chlorpromazine, rats could be protected against constraint ulcers, and even fish against fright. The rats no longer developed ulcers, and the tranquillized fish stayed in their bowl without any change of colour caused by modification of the chromatophores; on the contrary, they remained pale, thus indicating blocking of the hypophyseal functions.

However, when I looked under the microscope at the hypothalamus of all these animals, in spite of the beneficial action of the neuroleptics and tranquillizers on their behaviour, I noticed the absence of the Gomori secretion granules, which, in spite of the drugs, had either been emptied into the hypophysis or their secretion had dried up.

Only one substance stopped the emptying and disappearance of the Gomori secretions. This was meclofenoxate.

From meclofenoxate to the mysterious Dr Polis

It was chiefly to talk about meclofenoxate that I had come to Varenna. This was a product my wife had synthesized in Paul Rumpf's laboratory at the National Scientific Research Centre. Meclofenoxate was a derivative of a plant hormone with particularly curious actions.

This substance easily crossed the cerebral barrier, augmented the reaction of the cerebral cortex to adrenaline, diminished and regulated the effects of hunger and thirst, and counteracted diabetes induced by alloxane. In old guinea pigs, whose nerve cells were discoloured by age pigments (lipofuscin pigments), administration of meclofenoxate cleared the cells, which regained an appearance of youth. Furthermore, meclofenoxate had mysteriously enabled neurosurgeons to rescue a few patients from more or less profound comas.

What I wanted to say at Varenna was that meclofenoxate was also the only product that could block Gomori secretions in the hypothalamus and prevent their emptying into the hypophysis.

After my lecture, I answered many questions put by my colleagues about the details of my experiments and the verification of my results. Nearly all the participants were agreed over the functions of the hypothalamus, and the localization of essential affective instincts in this region. One particularly attentive listener had followed my contribution, and this was my hotel neighbour, the mysterious Dr Polis, who had been introduced to me on the night of my arrival at Varenna.

During the break that followed our discussions, we went out into the gardens to chat on the paths, leaning our elbows on the balconies which overlooked the lake, or sitting on the stone seats of the landing stage. Dr Polis came up to me soon after my talk.

'I was very interested in what you have told us. I would like to experiment with your meclofenoxate. Could you send me some samples to the USA?'

I answered that this was possible, but it was a product that was to be patented by the CNRS, and the French state, and that I would have to know beforehand where the product would be going and the use which would be made of it.

Dr Polis seemed a little embarrassed by my questions.

'There are two ways round it,' he said. 'Either I have you asked by my government for a sample of meclofenoxate, and this would be through more official channels, but it would mean waiting at least two or three months for me to be able to experiment with the product. Or else you trust me, and you send ten or twenty grams of it directly to Professor Schmidt at the University of Pennsylvania, and he would pass it on to me.'

I was a little irritated by all the mystery with which Dr Polis surrounded himself. I spoke about it with Seymour Kety, who had once worked with Schmidt at Philadelphia. He confirmed to me that Dr Polis had been specially recommended by the US Office of Naval Research as a researcher of great value who was interested in important problems connected with neurochemistry. That was all he knew. On the other hand, he encouraged me to use the way recommended by Polis of sending the meclofenoxate to Professor Schmidt.

'If Schmidt passes on the product to Polis, this is an official channel; you need have no fear over what use will be made of the product. In any case, I will be able to speak about it to Professor Schmidt.'

I shall long remember those June days at Varenna. Our discussions on nerve structures in the big cool rooms of the Villa Monastero, alternating with breaks when we went out to chat. We were served tea or coffee under a bower where there were stone seats and a table under the foliage.

One afternoon, Professor Di Mattei, from Rome, and Daniel Bovet got an innkeeper to bring some cold white wine in a large flask, which we drank in blue terracotta cups. Varenna was truly the dream spot for talking about the limbic brain, the hypothalamus, where all the seeds of our anguishes were waiting in ambush, lurking and menacing.

On returning to Paris, I sent Dr Polis the samples of meclofenoxate he had asked me for. Forty-five days later, I received a letter from him suggesting I should visit him at a research centre in Johnsville, near Philadelphia. It was an official invitation from the US Office of Naval Research. I was going to Canada and the USA in September; I accepted Dr Polis's invitation.

From the world's to the astronauts' anguish

A sensory deprivation room is a chamber with black walls and smooth, padded, soundproofed partitions. In this enclosure an individual is left alone in complete darkness, with no object, no food, nothing that could stimulate any of the five senses. Then, one observes—or rather the individual experiencing it observes and reports—the ensuing sensations. In this exceptionally abnormal situation, hallucinatory reactions some times develop, and often there is uncontrollable anguish.

At the opposite extreme, there can be brightness, flashes of light, lamps, noise, hustle and bustle, disruption, life, incessant movement of people and machines; in this chaos, slapped in the face by propaganda and publicity, knocked senseless by the mass media, deafened by loud vibrations, sickened or sated by the abundance of worldly food, someone, in the streets of New York or Paris, just as in a sensory deprivation chamber, can likewise know anguish, anxiety and the fear of living.

September 1960

The train journey from New York to Philadelphia seemed short to me. On the platform at Philadelphia there were few people. Black porters put our luggage down on the platform. My wife tugged at my arm, and I turned around; a man in a uniform, with a peaked cap on which a badge could be made out, held out at arm's length a placard on which 'Dr and Mrs J. E. Thuillier' was written. He took care of our luggage and accompanied us to a long Cadillac where we took our seats.

Our peaked-capped guide got into the front of the icily air-conditioned car, sitting next to the driver. Two motorcycle escorts flanked our vehicle, and we went off to the sound of sirens, alerting the whole neighbourhood.

We crossed through the suburbs of Philadelphia, then through an area of less dense development. After a trip of about forty minutes we reached Johnsville, stopping at a wire-netting fence with guardrooms.

We had to show our passports, which were carefully examined, together with the letters of invitation from Dr Polis and those of the Johnsville US Naval Air Development Center. We were photographed, and a few minutes later we attached labels to our coats with our names and identity photographs.

Back in the car, we drove on for several kilometres, alongside a strange concrete road along where in several places cylindrical vehicles were standing. The car finally stopped in front of a building where about ten people were gathered on some steps. Dr Polis left the group and came to meet us. We climbed up the steps with him, and he introduced all the staff of his laboratory to us.

Right up to the moment when we met again in the auditorium of the research centre, I still did not know what had earned us this official welcome at Johnsville. Dr Polis explained to my wife and me that we were in a research centre of the Navy, where all the phenomena to which humans would be submitted when launched into space were being studied. The machine on a special track that we had seen in the camp enclosure was a rocket-powered train capable of achieving massive acceleration, as could the centrifuge for pilots that we were going to visit and which could give speeds equal to and greater than those of the rockets which would take up future astronauts.

'The problem which I have the task of studying,' Polis told me, 'is to protect the body against the phenomena of high acceleration, which, at the launch of high-speed rockets, can paralyse the astronaut's nervous system and cause disastrous accidents.'

Smiling, he added, 'You have, without knowing it, helped me greatly in my work, and I am keen to show you what we have found, thanks to you and the meclofenoxate which Madame Thuillier has synthesized. This is why we are happy to welcome you here today.'

Dr Polis, in the midst of his collaborators, then explained the details of his research to us. His essential problem was to find the reasons leading to death during acceleration, and ways of avoiding this.

Acceleration, as everybody knows, is the increase in speed per unit of time. When a body is dropped from a certain height it falls towards the ground, pulled by the earth's force of attraction (gravity), whose acceleration is represented by the letter g (an acceleration of 9.81 metres per second per second). When a rocket is launched into orbit around the earth, it, and its payload, are subject to accelerations several times this value.

Now, if a living organism is progressively subjected to increasing multiples of g, problems ranging from respiratory difficulty to loss of consciousness and death are encountered, either immediately, or after a few hours or even days later.

For his experiments, Bernard Polis submitted white rats to progressive acceleration, up to 18g. For this he used the large centrifuge, in the cabin of which, instead of astronauts, special wire-mesh cages were placed containing rats. Then the machine was set going to reach a desired acceleration for a chosen length of time.

At 18g, all the rats died. Of course, there was no question of submitting the first astronauts in the Mercury programme to such accelerations, but Dr Polis needed to find out what caused death by acceleration in the rats, and to try to protect them.

First, he noticed that physical shock was not the cause, because being well protected and immobilized in wire-netting boxes, the rats did not suffer any damage to their organs. The heart and blood vessels stood up to it. Death came indirectly from the brain; and after many experiments Dr Polis found that death came from disorders resulting from anarchic functioning of the hypophysis.

In rats subjected to hyperacceleration, Polis had tried all the drugs in the world that could have a 'checking' effect on the hypophysis. Of course he had tried the neuroleptics, the tranquillizers, and the antidepressants; but nothing countered the shock of acceleration.

The only way to protect the animals was by carrying out ablation of the hypophysis. All hypophysectomized rats stood up perfectly well to accelerations, even above 18g. Clearly there was no question of removing the astronauts' hypophyses, Polis had hung on to the idea of acting indirectly on this gland at the base of the brain. It was in the hope of learning something new about the limbic brain that he had come to Varenna. The action of meclofenoxate had interested him, because he thought of blocking the hypothalamus secretion with the product, thus avoiding the rupture of the hypophyseal barrage, which led to biological cataclysm and death through acceleration.

'Up till today,' he told me, 'you have found the only product known to reduce the percentage of deaths due to acceleration.'

He showed me the results of his experiments, which I reproduced a few months later in Paris, at the Air Force test centre, directed by General Grognot. With Roger Roudier, Jean L'Huillier and R. Marchadier, I was able to demonstrate that in the presence of meclofenoxate, the Gomori secretions remained blocked in the hypothalamus during strong accelerations, without flooding the hypophysis, thus achieving secretory regulation of the whole base of the brain.

My meeting in the USA with Dr Polis was friendly and warm. He explained to me the reserve he had shown at the time of our first meeting at Varenna, and which he justified by the discretion that had to surround aerospace programmes. At our departure the same ceremony of military in uniforms, and outriders with sirens sounding, accompanied us to the airport.

In Washington I had another warm welcome from Joel Elkes in his hospital department, and the next day from Seymour Kety, director of research at the National Institute of Mental Health at Bethesda. In the sumptuous laboratories of this extraordinary institute, which collected Nobel prizes, I again met my friends Julius Axelrod, Paul MacLean and Roger McDonald.

For several years all these men were, like me, studying the structure, organization and physiology of this kilogram of soft, greasy, whitish material that our cranium encloses. We have examined the millions of cells that make it up, and the mysterious substances that impregnate it, circulate through it, and assure its function by regulating its mechanism. With many others we have already succeeded, thanks to new chemical molecules, in restoring disrupted circuits and putting forward effective medication. The discoveries achieved justify the official encouragement and large funds that have made it possible to equip our laboratories.

After Washington, I ended my American tour in New York, where I met some other psychopharmacology pioneers: Paul Hoch, director of mental health services for New York State, one of the first American psychiatrists to have used hallucinogens in experimental psychiatry—we had just elected him president of the CINP—and Herman Denber, a specialist in studies on mescaline and the first American experimenter with the neuroleptics, chlorpromazine and haloperidol.

As for Nathan S. Kline, he invited me to visit his department and his laboratory at Rockland State Hospital, where he had developed his work on reserpine, iproniazid and the MAOIs. At the end of the visit, with his customary humour, he told me that after the hors-d'oeuvre of psychotropic drugs he was going to treat me to an American dinner. In a New Jersey restaurant, on a warm September evening, we enjoyed an enormous guaranteed and labelled steak, accompanied by an American Roquefort salad and washed down with a sparkling red iced burgundy. When we parted that night, Kline pointed out the sky and the stars to me:

'It is beautiful, the night,' he said, 'but what a pity it makes us sleep. What a waste of time! All those hours frittered away. Genghis Khan and his troops only slept three hours a night. You'll have to find a drug which lets us rest our cerebral cells without going to sleep!'

In the aircraft that took me back to Paris I could not stop thinking of all these meetings with fellow doctors and researchers who, like me, had pulled all the strings and tried in every way to get neurochemistry and psychopharmacology on stage. And I was not indifferent to the thought that I had myself been amongst the actors who had taken part in creating this spectacle.

Of all these meetings, my visit to Philadelphia and Polis's welcome had been more than a reward. I could not get out of my mind visions of the science-fiction atmosphere where, within the framework of the Mercury programme, the launching of the astronaut John Glenn, in the first orbital flight by an American around the earth, was being prepared. At Johnsville I had been through the air-conditioned precincts of laboratories automated to the extreme, walked along the rails of the rocket-train propulsion ramps, and been inside the amphitheatres where the huge centrifuge arms spun round. Everywhere there were men dressed in tunics, light-coloured uniforms, boiler suits of scientifically treated nylon, specially designed protective masks, moving about in an organized and calculated manner with no unnecessary hustle, in the most peaceful manner. Despite this calmness, they also were going to be subjected to anguish, to a violent wrench from their peace; they still had to be protected and shielded from anxiety, as well as from the serious problems that could strike them down in such a dangerous enterprise.

All this was very different from the atmosphere of noise, rage and anguish into which I had been plunged ten years before, to resolve other problems. It was, nevertheless, in that other world of wards of mentally ill patients, and in the mental distress of depressed patients, that I had tried to find something better than the gag and the straitjacket to overpower mental illness. It was the sight of sinister daily processions of mentally ill patients, clothed in thick blue cloth and dragging their unlaced shoes over the gravel of the courtyards, that stopped me accepting chemical or electric shock muggings, and surgical ploughing up of the brain, as final.

Assuredly we have not yet found the 'mental stability pill' that could bring back those lost souls who cultivate hatred, violence and evil criminal instincts, into the heart of the community. Although psychopharmacology has not resolved everything in mental medicine, at least it has, in ten years, removed the straitjacket from agitated patients, released most patients with delirium from the asylum, and consoled those with depression and melancholia.

For the world's anguish, if we have been able to reveal its hiding place, we still need to perfect the tranquillizer that will succeed, if not in driving it out, at least in suffocating it in its den.

In spite of this, some still think that reason is everybody's madness, and that it is better to go along with this folly, rather than combat it with drugs, which are only chemical straitjackets in which freedom is imprisoned. For these anti-establishment people, it is perhaps easy to go into raptures over the poetry of other folk's delirium, the beauty of desperate clamours, and the feats of delirious imaginations; but when an ill wind blows insurmountable sadness and the will to die into poor souls, what help will there be to get them through the squall?

The sympathetic ear of the doctor or psychotherapist attentive to their complaints and sympathizing with their distress will bring them helpful support, in time; but why deny them the comfort and peace that a few beneficial elixirs can give them right away? Stopping the tumult of their thoughts, taking their anguish away, and breaking up obsessive delirium is what the new drugs can achieve. And even if this appeasement were only artificial or temporary, it would still have the merit of helping people to go on living.

And so, tomorrow . . .

Paris, 29 September 2080

Now, I must reply to those who decline to remain hungry, to those who always want to know more, who want to be acquainted with the prospects for the future, and which dishes will be served to them at the table of the blessed, which pills they will swallow when entering the church of the mentally ill in the twenty-first century.

The progress of psychiatric treatment, which I have described from the time of the colonel with the golden head, through to the moods of the NASA astronauts, may give the idea that tomorrow it will be possible to do anything, change everything—states of mind, consciousness, delirium and brains alike. Many wish to know how the history of mental illness in the ultramodern age will be written, and what the psychopharmacology and the psychiatry of an 'applied general relativity' will be.

'You certainly have a few ideas. You know what treatments are in use. Who will be able to foresee what it will be possible to do better than you?'

I have always refused to respond to those who want medical science fiction. But one pretentious person said to me, 'What has been is less important to me than what is; what is, less important than what could be, and will be.'

I then took the fly, because the sentence was not his own. I have known it for a long time; a quotation from Gide. It was a good deal longer. I have completed it:

'I too get muddled between possible and future. I think that everything possible endeavours to be, and that everything that could be, will be if man gives his help.'

So I, too, have wished to make an attempt like H. G. Wells, Jules Verne or H. P. Lovecraft. Since you would like to know, listen . . .

You see him, this deviant; this mentally ill patient of the future has been spotted by the continuous monitoring of the machines, which have not been any help to him because he despised them. He no longer knows how to use his magnetic identity or his internal codes; his directives, at the terminals at his workplace and home have been analysed without his knowing and found to be conflicting. His social, family and intimate, even sexual, behaviour, under sensor surveillance, has caused interference with his personal schedule. His mood, melancholic or too excited, is represented in the programming by rises or falls in his graphs, which have reached the warning levels. So, whether he likes it or not, he now stands before the Grand Inquisitor.

The Grand Inquisitor is the Machine and the doctor, or the Doctor and the machine; I cannot distinguish in my crystal ball. I would like to have done without a psychiatrist in this clairvoyance, but one is there, flanked by the biologist, the biochemist and the surgeon, who are still indispensable to provide, program, and analyse the data on the machines.

The room is not large, but quiet and air-conditioned. The suspect, settled in front of a console, is made to rest his hands on an analysing plate which carries out painless sampling of blood from the fingertips. All the biological constants are checked in a few seconds and stored in spare memory.

Behind the console a male or female doctor is sitting. The filtered voice is sexless, and difficult to distinguish from that of the robots. A few brief questions are put to the patient, for the whole history of his life and of his antecedents and descendants is already stored in his identity card. The Grand Inquisitor is just looking for the analysis of his verbal and behavioural reactions. Then the suspected deviant will pronounce a few sentences collected in acoustic cups, and even if he says nothing, the silence and negativism will be interpreted by the thousands of optical scanners that monitor expression, the general attitude and the choice of movements.

That will be all; the Grand Inquisitor machine will match the memory data with the patient's card code, the blood analysis results and the behavioural assessment. The diagnosis and treatment will come out in coded prescriptions. These prescriptions will be of three kinds, with gradual adjustments according to the severity of the disorders:

- restoration of mood equilibrium with chemotherapeutic implants;
- structural modification of cerebral zones with active intracerebral probes;
- mental restructuring after dissolution–reconstruction of disrupted psyche.

The three procedures are autoregulated by miniaturized computers incorporated under the skin of the chest, and accessible to control from the terminals of the Grand Inquisitor's central computer.

Psychoanalytic treatment has disappeared; it no longer has any purpose. Out of curiosity, portraits of Freud have been kept in comfortable rooms where, as a hobby, nostalgic people with nothing to do whisper their little secrets into the electronic ears of computers that are droning like sleeping analysts. At the entrance to these rooms, an automatic checkpoint only lets through those who pay for the 'right of confession', which in this particular case cannot be paid for with a credit card, but only by slipping a golden sovereign into the machine.

For millions of individuals, the tranquillizer implants ensure gradual and long-term diffusion of the active ingredients. Their concentrations are adjusted by 'passive guidance', using three gyrostatic systems ensuring the autonomy of the personality; the subject's moods cannot be accidentally upset from endogenous or exogenous causes. All the psychotropic chemical substances now cross the famous blood–brain barrier, which was formerly often impenetrable by foreign molecules. A kind of 'missile carrier' has been discovered, a vegetative hormone that opens the barrier for molecules with which it has been combined.

Lithium has at last given up its secret. The resonances relevant to specific receptors have been found. The problem of permanent microcrystals has been resolved, and once for everybody, a charge of metal circulating in the blood ensures permanent mental equilibrium. Furthermore, the diffraction pattern scale of lithium has been reconstructed on inert neurotransmitters and their application to pre- and post-synaptic receptor sites makes regulation of manic states possible as well as that of melancholia attacks. The most spectacular consequence of this discovery is that the use of tricyclic and MAOI antidepressants and also the major tranquillizers in manic-depressive syndromes has come to an end. The whole mood is now regulated by lithium salt diffraction. As regards lithium blood level measurements, patients are no longer submitted to this, the single charge of permanent crystals acting as a satellite network.

For severe delirium, psychoses and schizophrenias, molecular psychopharmacology has worked out made-to-measure neuroleptics, which reach the diencephalic centres in no time, before permeating the cerebral cortex. In spite of all the progress made, however, the origin of the major psychoses is still unknown. They are treated by total mental dissolution with massive doses of LSD administered in the form of crystalline implants inserted into the submaxillary glands. Then, when the brain shows complete affective-sensory emptying, psychomotor and sensory-affective images are reconstructed with the help of programs predetermined with the Grand Inquisitor's logistic calculators.

Strange things have began to disturb the most recent programs. The localizations of the cerebral mental zones associated with disorders of the body image have established unquestionable indices following which schizophrenia and most of the non-degenerative major psychoses will be inscribed and programmed outside the brain and positioned on meridians analogous to those drawn by Chinese acupuncturists. Thus the eight hundred bilateral points of acupuncture of the twelve principal meridians have been combined in their psychological implications by machines. And so a surprising conclusion has been reached: 'Psychological energy which always, and successively, runs in two Yin meridians, then two Yang meridians, always makes its specific mutation at the distal extremities of these vectors, that is to say at the level of the hands and feet.'

This information will not stop schizophrenia being treated by a combination of the two programs, one controlling the distribution of drugs with intracerebral probes, and the other mobilizing the re-educational impulses with electrodes implanted in the caudate nucleus and body of Luys.

All patients, who have their computers, in miniaturized form, inserted under the skin of their armpits, will from then on be able to check them with an intradermal relay contact at their waist.

Asylums will disappear. Parks and village treatment clubs for therapeutic trials will replace them. Some historic buildings like Charenton and Bonneval will be scheduled and opened as historic monuments. No longer would anybody claim the right to mental illness. Anti-psychiatry would disappear, like psychiatry itself, which would be absorbed into medical neurology and human psychological science, without anyone being able to discern the dividing line. Madness has become everybody's reason.

In spite of all the progress achieved, with some steadfastly incurable cases, brain grafts were envisaged. At the Weizmann Institute in Israel, David Samuel had transplanted the frontal area of the brain of a lizard in the 1960s. This time, the object was to replace the whole brain, as the American White had done around the same time with dogs and monkeys. But the task proved impossible.

The brain is a soft mass that is difficult to dissect, difficult to detach, and difficult to handle and transport. It is like a pastry-cook's sculpture in butter; you cannot pick it up with your hands or an instrument, for it falls apart, loses its shape, and slides away. It must be moved with its support, its base or its container. For the human brain the best thing was to keep the container—in other words; the head.

The first head was grafted on 24 June 2021 at the Defence hospital in Dr Vercors's department. It was Jean Druche, a patient who was still young but who was suffering from a progressive cerebral atrophy called Pick's disease. Within a body physically in excellent condition, Jean Druche's brain had gradually sunk into dementia. Lost in time and space, forgetting his words, how to use the most commonplace articles, and make the most elementary movements, Druche was no more than a puppet who fell apart a little more every day. Luck had it that Paul Muller, who had a Nobel prize for physics, was admitted to the same hospital for a heart transplant. This scientist was one of the last survivors from the thalidomide drama—the drug that had caused pregnant women to give birth to babies without arms and sometimes without legs.

Paul Muller resembled the Little Mermaid in Copenhagen, but with two small stumps for arms under his shoulders. His head, in contrast, was magnificent, with penetrating eyes, and the clear features of a man who lives for science. He was asked if he would agree to give his brain to Jean Druche in the event that the thoracic implantation of an artificial heart–lung was not successful.

'Since infancy, I have walked with artificial legs, my arms are levers, and my hands are articulated claws. Now I am going to have one more piece of mechanism in my chest. It is I,' he said, 'who am asking for Jean Druche's body for Paul Muller's head.'

Professors Vercors and Toful agreed, and during the night of 23–24 June, the operation began.

It was not known exactly whose head was taken off first—something which was very important later on.

The section was made at the level of the thyroid isthmus in front, and the sixth cervical vertebra behind. The artery and vein sutures were delicate because one wanted to keep Muller's thyroid, whereas anatomically it is Druche's that should have been transplanted. The problem of connecting up the muscles and nerves and bones was sorted out without difficulty. At the level of the two cut ends of the cervical spinal cord, Levon Matinian implants were used—the Armenian scientist who in 1976 had grown the first spinal cord.

Everything went well. As is known, with the brain, spinal cord and nerves, there is practically no rejection problem. For the other tissues, Druche's body and Muller's head had been treated with injections of immuno-strial substances, to avoid these sorts of reactions.

Fifteen days after the operation, Druche-Muller, or Muller-Druche, was talking, eating, and standing in front of a blackboard with a stick of chalk in his hand, giving a new demonstration of restricted relativity.

In the big amphitheatre at the Defence hospital, where Professors Vercors and Toful were presenting their operation case, two women were creating a scene. These were the respective wives of Druche and Muller, who were each wanting to take her husband home.

A police officer came to put an end to this argument with an arrest warrant relating to Jean Druche being guilty of homicide on the person of Paul Muller. For, legal death only being recognized after brain death, Jean Druche, with the complicity of the surgeons, was accused of having appropriated a still-living brain, by stealing the healthy brain of a dying body. So he had killed Paul Muller.

At the trial, the lawyer who pleaded for Jean Druche's body asked the lawyer of Muller's head to defend his client, maintaining that Druche had made him a present of his body. The counsel for the prosecution, who could no longer demand Druche's guilty head, which he confused with Muller's, got muddled up in his summing up for the prosecution. Muller-Druche was acquitted. The public prosecutor's department appealed and Druche-Muller was condemned. On appeal, the case was dismissed . . . here I shall stop conjuring up these things so as not to worry Justice, let my neighbours sleep, and tiptoe out before they wake up.

Index